Morbus anglicus: or, The anatomy of consumptions Containing the nature, causes, subject, progress, change, signes, prognosticks, preservatives; and several methods of curing all consumptions, coughs, and spitting of blood. (1666)

Gideon Harvey

Morbus anglicus: or, The anatomy of consumptions Containing the nature, causes, subject, progress, change, signes, prognosticks, preservatives; and several methods of curing all consumptions, coughs, and spitting of blood.
Harvey, Gideon, 1640?-1700?
With three final contents leaves.
Copy cataloged has considerable print show-through; tightly bound with slight loss of print.
[8], 250, [6] p.
London : printed for Nathaniel Brook at the Angel in Cornhil, 1666.
Wing (2nd ed.) / H1070
English
Reproduction of the original in the Bodleian Library

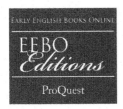

Early English Books Online (EEBO) Editions

Imagine holding history in your hands.

Now you can. Digitally preserved and previously accessible only through libraries as Early English Books Online, this rare material is now available in single print editions. Thousands of books written between 1475 and 1700 and ranging from religion to astronomy, medicine to music, can be delivered to your doorstep in individual volumes of high-quality historical reproductions.

We have been compiling these historic treasures for more than 70 years. Long before such a thing as "digital" even existed, ProQuest founder Eugene Power began the noble task of preserving the British Museum's collection on microfilm. He then sought out other rare and endangered titles, providing unparalleled access to these works and collaborating with the world's top academic institutions to make them widely available for the first time. This project furthers that original vision.

These texts have now made the full journey -- from their original printing-press versions available only in rare-book rooms to online library access to new single volumes made possible by the partnership between artifact preservation and modern printing technology. A portion of the proceeds from every book sold supports the libraries and institutions that made this collection possible, and that still work to preserve these invaluable treasures passed down through time.

This is history, traveling through time since the dawn of printing to your own personal library.

Initial Proquest EEBO Print Editions collections include:

Early Literature

This comprehensive collection begins with the famous Elizabethan Era that saw such literary giants as Chaucer, Shakespeare and Marlowe, as well as the introduction of the sonnet. Traveling through Jacobean and Restoration literature, the highlight of this series is the Pollard and Redgrave 1475-1640 selection of the rarest works from the English Renaissance.

Early Documents of World History

This collection combines early English perspectives on world history with documentation of Parliament records, royal decrees and military documents that reveal the delicate balance of Church and State in early English government. For social historians, almanacs and calendars offer insight into daily life of common citizens. This exhaustively complete series presents a thorough picture of history through the English Civil War.

Historical Almanacs

Historically, almanacs served a variety of purposes from the more practical, such as planting and harvesting crops and plotting nautical routes, to predicting the future through the movements of the stars. This collection provides a wide range of consecutive years of "almanacks" and calendars that depict a vast array of everyday life as it was several hundred years ago.

Early History of Astronomy & Space

Humankind has studied the skies for centuries, seeking to find our place in the universe. Some of the most important discoveries in the field of astronomy were made in these texts recorded by ancient stargazers, but almost as impactful were the perspectives of those who considered their discoveries to be heresy. Any independent astronomer will find this an invaluable collection of titles arguing the truth of the cosmic system.

Early History of Industry & Science

Acting as a kind of historical Wall Street, this collection of industry manuals and records explores the thriving industries of construction; textile, especially wool and linen; salt; livestock; and many more.

Early English Wit, Poetry & Satire

The power of literary device was never more in its prime than during this period of history, where a wide array of political and religious satire mocked the status quo and poetry called humankind to transcend the rigors of daily life through love, God or principle. This series comments on historical patterns of the human condition that are still visible today.

Early English Drama & Theatre

This collection needs no introduction, combining the works of some of the greatest canonical writers of all time, including many plays composed for royalty such as Queen Elizabeth I and King Edward VI. In addition, this series includes history and criticism of drama, as well as examinations of technique.

Early History of Travel & Geography

Offering a fascinating view into the perception of the world during the sixteenth and seventeenth centuries, this collection includes accounts of Columbus's discovery of the Americas and encompasses most of the Age of Discovery, during which Europeans and their descendants intensively explored and mapped the world. This series is a wealth of information from some the most groundbreaking explorers.

Early Fables & Fairy Tales

This series includes many translations, some illustrated, of some of the most well-known mythologies of today, including Aesop's Fables and English fairy tales, as well as many Greek, Latin and even Oriental parables and criticism and interpretation on the subject.

Early Documents of Language & Linguistics

The evolution of English and foreign languages is documented in these original texts studying and recording early philology from the study of a variety of languages including Greek, Latin and Chinese, as well as multilingual volumes, to current slang and obscure words. Translations from Latin, Hebrew and Aramaic, grammar treatises and even dictionaries and guides to translation make this collection rich in cultures from around the world.

Early History of the Law

With extensive collections of land tenure and business law "forms" in Great Britain, this is a comprehensive resource for all kinds of early English legal precedents from feudal to constitutional law, Jewish and Jesuit law, laws about public finance to food supply and forestry, and even "immoral conditions." An abundance of law dictionaries, philosophy and history and criticism completes this series.

Early History of Kings, Queens and Royalty

This collection includes debates on the divine right of kings, royal statutes and proclamations, and political ballads and songs as related to a number of English kings and queens, with notable concentrations on foreign rulers King Louis IX and King Louis XIV of France, and King Philip II of Spain. Writings on ancient rulers and royal tradition focus on Scottish and Roman kings, Cleopatra and the Biblical kings Nebuchadnezzar and Solomon.

Early History of Love, Marriage & Sex

Human relationships intrigued and baffled thinkers and writers well before the postmodern age of psychology and self-help. Now readers can access the insights and intricacies of Anglo-Saxon interactions in sex and love, marriage and politics, and the truth that lies somewhere in between action and thought.

Early History of Medicine, Health & Disease

This series includes fascinating studies on the human brain from as early as the 16th century, as well as early studies on the physiological effects of tobacco use. Anatomy texts, medical treatises and wound treatment are also discussed, revealing the exponential development of medical theory and practice over more than two hundred years.

Early History of Logic, Science and Math

The "hard sciences" developed exponentially during the 16th and 17th centuries, both relying upon centuries of tradition and adding to the foundation of modern application, as is evidenced by this extensive collection. This is a rich collection of practical mathematics as applied to business, carpentry and geography as well as explorations of mathematical instruments and arithmetic; logic and logicians such as Aristotle and Socrates; and a number of scientific disciplines from natural history to physics.

Early History of Military, War and Weaponry

Any professional or amateur student of war will thrill at the untold riches in this collection of war theory and practice in the early Western World. The Age of Discovery and Enlightenment was also a time of great political and religious unrest, revealed in accounts of conflicts such as the Wars of the Roses.

Early History of Food

This collection combines the commercial aspects of food handling, preservation and supply to the more specific aspects of canning and preserving, meat carving, brewing beer and even candy-making with fruits and flowers, with a large resource of cookery and recipe books. Not to be forgotten is a "the great eater of Kent," a study in food habits.

Early History of Religion

From the beginning of recorded history we have looked to the heavens for inspiration and guidance. In these early religious documents, sermons, and pamphlets, we see the spiritual impact on the lives of both royalty and the commoner. We also get insights into a clergy that was growing ever more powerful as a political force. This is one of the world's largest collections of religious works of this type, revealing much about our interpretation of the modern church and spirituality.

Early Social Customs

Social customs, human interaction and leisure are the driving force of any culture. These unique and quirky works give us a glimpse of interesting aspects of day-to-day life as it existed in an earlier time. With books on games, sports, traditions, festivals, and hobbies it is one of the most fascinating collections in the series.

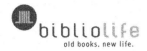

The BiblioLife Network

This project was made possible in part by the BiblioLife Network (BLN), a project aimed at addressing some of the huge challenges facing book preservationists around the world. The BLN includes libraries, library networks, archives, subject matter experts, online communities and library service providers. We believe every book ever published should be available as a high-quality print reproduction; printed on-demand anywhere in the world. This insures the ongoing accessibility of the content and helps generate sustainable revenue for the libraries and organizations that work to preserve these important materials.

The following book is in the "public domain" and represents an authentic reproduction of the text as printed by the original publisher. While we have attempted to accurately maintain the integrity of the original work, there are sometimes problems with the original work or the micro-film from which the books were digitized. This can result in minor errors in reproduction. Possible imperfections include missing and blurred pages, poor pictures, markings and other reproduction issues beyond our control. Because this work is culturally important, we have made it available as part of our commitment to protecting, preserving, and promoting the world's literature.

GUIDE TO FOLD-OUTS MAPS and OVERSIZED IMAGES

The book you are reading was digitized from microfilm captured over the past thirty to forty years. Years after the creation of the original microfilm, the book was converted to digital files and made available in an online database.

In an online database, page images do not need to conform to the size restrictions found in a printed book. When converting these images back into a printed bound book, the page sizes are standardized in ways that maintain the detail of the original. For large images, such as fold-out maps, the original page image is split into two or more pages

Guidelines used to determine how to split the page image follows:

• Some images are split vertically; large images require vertical and horizontal splits.
• For horizontal splits, the content is split left to right.
• For vertical splits, the content is split from top to bottom.
• For both vertical and horizontal splits, the image is processed from top left to bottom right.

Morbus Anglicus:
OR,
THE ANATOMY
OF
CONSUMPTIONS.

CONTAINING

The Nature, Caufes, Subject,
Progrefs, Change, Signes, Progno-
fticks, Prefervatives ; and feveral
Methods of *Curing* all *Confumptions*
Coughs, and *Spitting of Blood.*
With Remarkable Obfervations touching the
fame *DISEASES.*

To which are Added ,
Some brief Difcourfes of *Melancholy, Mad-*
nefs , and Diftraction occafioned by Love.

Together with certain new Remarques
touching the *Scurvy* and *Ulcers* of the *Lungs.*

The like never before publifhed.

By *GIDEON HARVEY,* M. D.

London, Printed for *Nathaniel Brook* at
the *Angel* in *Cornhil.* 1666.

Advertisement to the Reader

ADVERTISEMENT
TO THE
READER.

LEst my Reader's Phansie should be distemper'd with that common brain-disease of Jealousie, in calling to accompt the design of the Author, or the contents, and Phrase of his discourse, I shall do him kindness, and my self right, in preinforming his judgment to anticipate those too frequent injust censures, both of the one and the other; I mean of Authour and Treatize. What concerns the design; it's universally known, that many write out of an itching, or affectation of seeing their names

in

Advertisement to the Reader.

in Print; others out of an interest, or expectation of Praise, preferment, or profit; and but few out of a single and ingenuous intent, to benefit the publick, and promote Learning. That vain scope of the first rank is manifestly apparent in the texture of what they expose to view, being tracts, Translated, or Compiled out of several Collections, which at the best deserve no other denomination, than patcht or botcht pieces. Neither can they easily palliate their sordid drift, that disperse Books for their profit, which contain little else, than a rude and imperfect description of what the Title promises, taking only an occasion thence to inform their Reader with one half, and to prompt 'em to repair to the Authour to buy the other half; this we see, is the ordinary design of many of those Physick Authours, that have of late years throngd into the stage. But being conscious of the sincerity of my own thoughts in that particular, I am very apt believe, there's no ingenious person but will upon the least survey of these Medical remarques, construe them designed

Advertisement to the Reader.

signed for publick advantage; or else should sooner devote 'em to the flame, than his lecture. And to render this Discourse more universal, and accommodated to the meaner capacities, I was desired to explain every hard word and term of Art; whereto I readily yielded, by joining another vulgar word to it in Italique Letters, included in a Parenthesis; which method is only observed in the former part, where the Reader must acquaint himself with the said terms and obscure words to understand the latter. To those of a more polish'd intellect that pains will seem needless, and the explications nauseous; However they may without regret pass it by, since in the bulk of the work I have chiefly endevour'd to gratifie them with matters of greater importance, and have omitted such insertions, which generally in other tracts are far more displeasing. In the first place whatever any of the whole Catalogue of Authours Ancient or Modern have writ concerning Consumptions, they will find it plainly digested in a third part only of this Treatise; the remainder

Advertisement to the Reader.

mainder I have fill'd up with very remarkable observations, both Theoretick, and Practical, which I had abstracted from the Diseases of many hundreds in several parts of Europe. Moreover I imagine, I have detected several errours many have and do still harbour touching the nature and Causes of a Consumption; which I have likewise dissected into all its possible kinds or Species. I have been very frank in giving you my own Sentiment of the essence and the various causes of the Disease; and thereunto added the solution of several very necessary queries; and at last set down the most approve'd methods for preservation and cure, used in Italy, Germany, and France, by the most famous of Hermetical and Dogmatical Physicians. Besides this general dissertation, I have made particular reflections throughout the whole on that sort of Consumption, that's so Endemick to this City; and strictly inquired into those external causes, viz. dyet, motion, air, &c. which latter I find to act the greatest part in this Morbifique aggression; as my self
can

Advertisement to the Reader.

an particularly witness; for having passed
nt a few months within the Walls, I
oon apprehended an oppression on my Lungs,
vhich then for my health's sake gave me
ccasion to make search for the best air
about Town, which after a serious consult
vith my thoughts I concluded to be in
Hatton-Garden, whither I immediately
transported my self, and do find it the purest
and most serene Air that's about the
City. This by the way, to give you an
instance of the benefit redounding from the
change of air, though but to a small
distance. Moreover touching the contents
of this following Tract, you'l meet with
some no vulgar observations on Womens
Diseases, which since plainly delineated,
may bring my modesty into question among
such as are unacquainted with discourses
of that nature. To these I have nothing
more to say, than that I move within
my own Sphere, and have render'd my
self in expressions familiar to Physicians.
But one point more I must prevent your
probable censure in, that having declared
the evils of a Spermatick Plethory, my
drift

Advertisement to the Reader.

drift is not to exhort any to incontinency, that monster of vice, but to prevent the danger of it by a spare Dyet, Devout Life, or (for the last and desperate remedy) by Marriage.

THE
ANATOMY
OF
CONSUMPTIONS.

The Proem.

*C*Ontingent (accidental) Death
seems to be the sole, adæquate
(juftly fitting) object of popular Cou-
rage; but a neceffary and unavoidable
coffin ftrikes palenefs into the ftouteft
heart, and beyond all other fwifter
terribles, the lazy but fure paces of a
Confumption, which we obferve oft
willingly inclines thofe to imbrace vain

B   *pity,*

pity, whose resolution Fire nor Sword can relaxe. This so mortal an Enemy to humane life doth the more earnestly implore succour from Charitable Physicians, the ambition to which Character hath wrested these Medical (Physical) pages (leaves) from our lucubrations (night Studies.)

CHAP. I.

Of the Original, Contagion, and frequency of Consumptions.

IT's a great chance we find, to arrive to ones grave in this *English* Climate, without a smack of a Consumption, Death's direct doore to most *English* hard Students, Divines, Physicians, Philosophers, deep Lovers, Zelots in Religion, &c. *London's* Weekly Bills number deep in Consumptions; the same likewise proving inseparable accidents (*attendants*) to most of the other Diseases;

Difeafes;which inftances do evidently bring a Confumption under the notion of a *Pandemick*,or *Endemick*,or rather a *Vernacular* Difeafe (*a difeafe alwayes reigning in a Countrey*) to *England*; that is a common difeafe owing its rife to fome common external and perennal (*lafting all the year*) caufe of a Countrey ; as a Confumptive Air, or a Confumptive Dyet. *viz*. eating much Flefh, drinking Hopt drink, *&c*. And beyond this denomination the difeafe may not improperly be ftiled Epidemick (*popular,*) that is, furprizing many at a certain feafon of the year; as we may obferve Confumptions to be moft raging about the Spring and Fall, according to the dictate of the Divine old man(*Hippocrates,*) *Malum ver tabidis, itemq̃, autumnus.* that is , the Spring is bad for Confumptives, and fo is the Fall. And confidering withall its malignity and catching nature, it may be connumerated (numbred) with the worft of *Epidemicks* (*popular difeafes,*) fince next to the Plague, Pox, and Leprofy, it yeilds to none in point of Contagion (*catching*;) for it's no rare obfervation here in *England*, to fee a frefh coloured lufty young man yoak'd to a Confumptive Female (*Wife,*) and him foon after attending her to the Grave. Moreover nothing we find taints found Lungs fooner, than infpiring (*drawing in*) the breath of putrid(*ftinking and beginning to rot*) ulcer'd, or confumptive Lungs; many having fallen into Confumptions only by fmelling the breath or fpittle of Confumptives, others by drinking after them; and what is more, by wearing the Cloaths of Confumptives, though two years after they were left off.

The difeafe defcending frequently from Confumptive Parents to their Children, fpeaks it Hereditary (*gotten as it were by inheritance from ones Parents,*) infomuch that whole Families, fourcing (*defcended* from tabefyed (*confumed and dryed away*) progenitours (*anceftors,*) have all made their *Exits* (dyed) through Confumptions; and in that order and Sympathy of confanguinity (*near Relation,*) that I have heard of fix Brothers Parifians (*Inhabitants of* Paris) all expired of Confumptions exactly fix months one after another. Befides, I have
known

known feveral, Father and Son, Mother and Daughter, tabefyed (confumed) within Twelve months one of the other.

Moft contagious Maladies (catching difeafes) have their Original recorded, the Leprofie in the primitive generation of the Jews, the Pox in the year 1494. the Scurvy in 1495; but the Confumption o'retops them all in antiquity, that queftionlefs being the primitive difeafe before all others, which in all probability put a period (*end*) to our Protoplafts (*firft formed*) *Adam* and *Eve's* days; for they being diffeifed (*turn'd out*) of their moft happy feat Paradife, and fo far difcarded (*caft out*) out of Gods favour, could not but fall into a moft difmal, fad, and melancholique drooping, for the lofs of their happinefs, the occafional caufe and forerunner of a *Marcour*, or drying and withering of their flefh and radical moifture (*the deep oyly moifture of the parts,*) or otherwife they might have Spun the thred of their lives much longer, their principles of life being created in them to extend to an Eval duration (*lafting without end.*)

B 3   C H A P.

CHAP. II.

Of the various acceptions of Consumptions.

THe common chink, through which errors and erroneous opinions do and have flipt into the Scholaftique republique, to the endangering and enfoncing(drowning) of truth, is the too frequent mifapprehenfion of the name of a thing, which being underftood in one fenfe by me, and in another by you, muft neceffarily occafion us to difcrepate (*difagree*) in the thing it felf; and this certainly is the great caufe of fo many controverfies and difputes between the Learned, and fuch others as are equally ballanced in right reafon : now were not the mifconception of the name various between them, being confidered really rational, they could notbut agree in the thing it felf, or otherwife they could not be eftimated both rational. When my felf was a Student in the Univerfities,

fities, and oft being defired to oppofe *ex tempore*, did no more than wilfully mifapprehend the names of things contained in the queftion, and upon thofe falfe nominal mif-confceptions, could with the greateft eafe imaginable perform that task as long as I pleafed, and fo may you, or any man elfe. Being now confcious of the great errors and dangers, that may refult out of a mif-conception of the names of things, fhall fo much the more apply my endevours to a diftinct explanation (*explaining*) of the names of my Subject, which ufually are varioufly underftood. Phyficians in their Phyfical difcourfes, make ufe of feveral names, which are all tranflated into this one word of a *Confumption*, as if they bore no different fignifications ; fuch are *Phthifis Phthoe*, *Pye*, *Tabes*, *Morbus tabificus*, *Marcor*, *Marafmus*, a Marcid Feaver, an Hectick Feaver, and an *Atrophia*.

The firft denomination, to wit *Phthifis*, an *Athenian* word, is generally taken for any kind of an univerfal diminution (*leffening*) and colliquation (*melting*) of the body, which acception its Etymology (*derivation*)

tion) Φθίσις ἀπὸ τῦ Φθίνειν, *to confume*, implyes ; but fome are of opinion the word Φθίσις ought to be written Φθύσις with an υ, deriving it from Φθύειν *to fpit*.

Hippocrates 7. Aph. 16. by *Phthifis* (*Confumption*) intends only fuch a diminution or fhrinking of the Body, as follows incurable Ulcers of the Lungs, that are accompanyed with a fmall Feaver. *Cornelius Celfus* applyed the word *Phthifis* to thefe three Difeafes. 1. to an *Atrophia*, and in that fignification did *Ariftotle* alfo take it, when he wrot in 28. *Probl.* 1. that *Dionyfius* dyed of a *Phthifis*. 2. To an Ulcer of the Lungs. 3. To a *Cachexia* , or ill habit of body ; but the Greek Phyficians were wont to call any one φθινώδη; i. e. *Phthificus*, who was either grown lean only , or who was taken with a proper *Phthifis*, and confumed away; or who was naturally inclined to a proper *Phthifis*, namely by having a long Neck, a narrow Cheft or Breaft, Shoulders fticking out like wings, (whence they named fuch a one πτερυγώδης, that is, winged) a weak Brain, apt to fend down Rheums or Catarrhs, and weak Lungs, that are

are difpofed to receive Rheums and humours from the Brain. Laftly, *Phthifis* is
properly and ftrictly taken according to
Hipp. for a Confumption of the Body, following an incurable Ulcer of the Lungs, and
attended with an Hectick Feaver.

Phthoe is likewife an *Athenian* word,
importing a proper Confumption, occafioned by an Ulcer of the Lungs ; but *Galen* 5.
Met. 15. by *Phthoe* intends the fpitting of
blood.

Pye is by *Aretæus* (*lib.* 1. *de cauf. &
fign. diut.*) ufed for a proper Confumption.

Tabes is the Latin word refponding (an-
fwering) to *Phthifis,* and implyes the fame
proper and improper fignifications. *Hippocrates* makes mention of fix forts of *Tabes,*
or proper Confumptions: *viz.* firft *libr.* 2.
de Morb. he affirms that the body oft wafts
by reafon of a thick Phlegm, being retained
within the Lungs, and there putrefying ;
according to which fenfe he writes, that a
Diftillation in the Lungs is fuppurated
(*turn'd to matter*) in twenty days. 7. *Aph.*
38. The fecond he terms a Confumption
of the Kidneys. Thirdly, the word *Tabes*
is

is oft underftood by him for a Confumption
of the Lungs without being ulcerated , and
depending upon a hot and dry Diftemper
of the Lungs, or an *Hectick Feaver.*
Fourthly, by *Tabes* he doth alfo conceive a
Confumption of the Lungs with an Ulcer
and Hectick Feaver. Fifthly , *lib.* 2. *de
Morb.* he inferts another kind of *Tabes*,
which he calls a *Tabes Dorfalis*, or
Confumption of the back. Sixthly, 3. *Aph.*
10. *&* 13. he propofes two kinds of *Tabes*
or Confumptions , the one being a wafting
of the body, occafioned by any internal
caufe , the other happening through fome
Ulcer in the Lungs. *Morbus tabificus*
is a term expreffed by *Hippocrates* ,
denoting any kind of Extenuation or Confumption.

    Marcor , *five ex ægritudine Senectus,
feu ex Morbo Senium* , is an extreme
diminution or Confumption of the body,
following the extinction (quenching) of
the *Innate* (born and bred in us) heat, much
like to a tree , that's withered or dryed
away by excefs of heat, or length of time.
The faid *Marcour* may likewife be caufed
                        by

by Famine or over abstinence from food.
Read *Galen lib. de* Marcore.

A *Marasmus*, imports three significa-
tions, *viz.* 1. A Consumption following a
Feaver. 2. A Consumption or withering of
the body by reason of a natural extinction of
the native heat, which commonly happens
in those that dye of old Age. 3. An extenuation of the body, caused through an immoderate heat and driness of the parts,
which sort is common to young and old
folks. A *Marasmus* is otherwise distinguish'd
into true and false. The former is an equal
diminution of all the parts of the body ; the
latter is an extenuation (*shrinking*) of a
single part only ; as, the Stomach and Liver
are oft observed to be consumed or withered in those, that dye of an Hectick Feaver ;
the like extenuation doth frequently happen
to the breast, *Mesentery* (a thick Skin of
the Belly that tyes the Guts) *Colon, Jeju-
num*, (both names of Guts) and Kidneys ;
but the *Diaphragma* (the Midriffe , being
a thick Musculous Skin that separates the
breast from the Belly) is only exempted
from a *Marasmus*, or withering, because
that

that would necessarily intercept the breath, or occasion a Phrensie, before it could arrive to such a dryness. Lastly, a *Marcour* is either imperfect, tending to a greater withering, which is cureable; or perfect, that is an entire wasting of the body, excluding all means of Cure.

Febris Marasmodes, seu febris marcida, according to *Galen lib. de* Marcore *cap.* 5. is an equal withering or drying up of all the parts of the body, it's ordinarily a consequent of a burning colliquative (*melting*) Feaver, whereby the humours, grease, fat, and flesh of the body are melted, and afterwards flow into the capacity (*hollow*) of the Belly: The softer and moister parts being thus melted away, the Febril (*Feaverish*) heat continuing its adustion (*burning*) upon the dryer fleshy parts, changes into a *Marcid Feaver*, which said parts wasting gradually through an insensible evaporation of their subtiler particles, are at length dryed up into the hardness and toughness of Leather.

An Hectick Feaver implyes a two-fold sense. 1. It's taken for any confirm'd, fix'd, fix'd, and durable Feaver, admitting of no easie cure, or rather a Feaver that's grown *habitual*, in opposition to a Schetical *(superficial or moveable)* Feaver, which being but lately arrived is easily expelled, as a *Diary* or *Putrid Feaver.* 2. It's more generally understood for a Feaver in the solid parts, into whose Penetrails *(depth)* and essential principles insinuating, is there as it were planted or rooted, and consequently proves the most stubborn to Cure of all other Diseases. *What is meant by the solid parts and the Essential principles you may know in the next Chapter.*

An *Atrophy* is by some taken for a diminution of the body, for want of good and laudable nutriment *(food,)* which being rejected by the parts, must necessarily shrink for want of better nutriture. By others it's understood for a Consumption of the parts of the body, weakly, or depravately *(wrongly,)* or not at all attracting nutriment, whether it be good or bad, or insufficient in quantity. Lastly, it implyes a diminution of the body, happening by reason of some fault in the *Excretive*(expelling)

ling) *faculty* of the parts, excerning or evacuating more than neceſſary. Peruſe *Galen de Sympt. differ. cap.* 4. The ſaid Conſumption may alſo be ſuppoſed to arrive through fault of the Retentive *(retaining)* faculty of the parts, not retaining the nutritive *(nouriſhing)* humours long enough. Thus much for differencing thoſe terms, which otherwiſe might erroneouſly be taken for one and the ſame kind of Conſumption.

CHAP. III.

Of the Fundamental Principles, or Balſamick Mixture.

BEfore we make a further inroad into this Treatiſe, it will be material to acquaint my Reader with the ſenſe of theſe terms, which we have familiarly made uſe of throughout this diſcourſe, namely *Fundamental* or *Eſſential Principles, Eſſential* or *Balſamick* mixture, *Innate heat* and
Radical

Radical or *Balfamick moifture :* all thefe
though differing in words, import the fame
fignification, as we fhall now difcover to
you. In order to this, you are to take
notice, that an Infant in the Womb principally receives its firft conftitution or
generation from the Sperm (*or Seed*) of
its Father, injected (*caft into*) into the
Womb of its Mother, which (to wit the
Womb) contributes little elfe to it, than
the earth to the Seed, that's fhed or fown
in her, namely keeps the Seed clofe together, that the Spirits may not evaporate
(*fly out in vapours,*) cherifhes it by her own
Innate (*rooted and fix'd*) and *Influent* (fent
from the heart) heat and fpirits, thereby
ftirring, ftrengthening, and affifting the
fpirits of the Seed in the Womb, in forming
the parts of the Infant intended; and laftly,
tranfmits blood to the Seed to give the parts
fo formed an increafe. The Seed confifting
of a glutinous (*glewy*) or Balfamick (*thick
and cleaving like to a Balfam*) moifture,
and a turgency (*fulnefs*) of Spirits, difplays
it felf (being now thus inclofed and ftirred
in the Womb) into feveral parts of various
(*different*)

(*different*) figures and shapes, as, into a
Heart, Brain, Liver, Spleen, Arms, Legs, &c.
These parts being of a very small proportion, as formed out of a small quantity of
Seed, are no more than *Foundation Piles* of
the ensuing body; which are afterwards to
be increased and raised to a greater bulk,
by the affluent (*flowing to*) blood, that's
transmitted (*sent down*) out of the Mothers
body through proper Veins and Arteries
into the Womb, where it's glewed fast to
those said foundation (rather fundamental)
parts, and soon after assimilated or converted into flesh, and other *similar* substan-
ces, whereby I say every part grows bigger.

The Infant being thus arrived to a competent Mole (*bigness,*) makes its sally out
of the Womb, that's now grown too little
to give it any longer harbour; and having
thus passed the Streights, it's tossed into the
wide world, where it has got room enoug
to grow into its full dimension (measure,
which is performed by the daily ingestio
(*swallowing down*) of milk and other food
that's in a short time after digested int
blood which being diffused (*spread abroad*
throug

through the Arteries and Veins to all the parts of the body, is, as we inftanced before, agglutinated (*glewed*) to thofe upper parts, that were immediately agglutinated to the foundation parts in the Womb: and thus you fee the Infant grows bigger out of the Womb, by agglutinating one afflux of blood to another. Upon this premitted illuftration it's no hard task to exprefs to you the meaning of *Fundamental* or *Effential Principles*, which imply nothing elfe than the forementioned *Foundation parts.* So like-wife the *Effential* or *Balfamick mixture* denotes nothing but the Sperm or Seed, whereof the fundamental parts confift; and it's called *Balfamick mixture*, becaufe it's a glewy fpumous matter, mix'd with a great quantity of *Plaftick* fpirits (or fpirits of the Sperm, that form the fhape of the parts in the Womb) into the confiftence of a Balfam, and may not improperly be named Effential, from its conftituting the effence of the parts. The faid *Plaftick* fpirits are concomitated (*attended*) with a powerful heat, which is therefore denomi-nated (*named*) the *Innate heat* (or heat

C   bor:

born in us,) becaufe its rooted and fix'd in the fundamental parts, and is infeparable from them during life. The Balfamick moifture expreffes the glewy fpumous matter of the Sperm, which is termed *Radical*, or the root moifture, becaufe it's the root and foundation of all the parts of the body.

Finding you thus conducted through a fmooth way, we'll inftantly open a door, to give you paffage to a more abftrufe *(hidden,)* but pleafant fpeculation, *viz.* the manner of a proper and improper Confumption, together with the reafon of the incurability of the former, and facil *(eafie)* cure of the other. The Sanguin parts, that are fuperftructed *(built)* upon the faid Spermatick *(feedy,)* or rather Fundamental parts, out of the continual afflux *(flowing to)* of blood to them, may per-chance be wafted or diminifh one day for want of materials, namely blood, or by reafon of fome indifpofition or fault in the blood; the next day poffibly thofe defects of the blood may be fupplyed by a copious *(plentiful)* afflux of good blood, whereby the preceeding diminifh'd parts happen to re-
increaf

increafe. Which ebbing and flowing of the
parts may in no wife be cenfured a Confumption, improper or proper. But fuppofing the forementioned Confumption
fhould prove fo durable, as to abforb *(dry
up)* and extenuate *(diminifh)* the faid Sanguin parts to an extreme degree, it's evident, that the Fundamental parts muft
necéffarily come into danger; which being
once attaqued *(forcibly enter'd upon,)* and
confiderably confumed, the fuperftructure
*(or the whole body, that's built upon the
Fundamental parts,)* muft unavoidably fall
and come to ruine; which degree of Confumption we term a *proper Confumption,* as
obtaining its feat in the foundation of the
body, and admitting for the moft part of no
cure, or at leaft a very difficult one. We
may appofitely *(to our purpofe)* compare
this difcourfe of a proper and improperCon-
fumption to a decaying houfe, which though
decaying or falling away by lofing a roof,
or a wall, comes in no great danger; but
if neglected, the houfe begins to totter, and
continuates its rupture *(breach)* to the very
foundation, which once wafted or endam-

maged, the house muſt neceſſarily fall; and ſo the caſe ſtands with a ſuperficial or improper, and a fundamental or proper Conſumption of the body. So that as you'l read in the next enſuing Chapter, it's not every over-faſting, or over-labouring, or Phyſicking, that renders a man lean, and extenuates his parts, comes within the Sphere of a Conſumption, ſince ſuch an impair is ſoon rectifyed again; but as I inferred in the 4. Chapter, it's a durable and ſomewhat an habitual extenuation (*or waſting*) of the Sanguin or Fleſhy parts, that are not eaſily reduced to their priſtine (*old*) conſtitution, by reaſon of ſome habitual fault or diſeaſe of an Entrail, moving directly to the Fundamental parts, where it may effect a perfect Conſumption.

CHAP.

CHAP. IV.

Of the nature of a Confumption in general.

THe word *Confumption* being applicable to a proper and improper, or true and Baftard Confumption, requires from us a Generiŝal (*general*) defcription, quadrate (*fitting*) to both. So that a Confumption in that refpeŝt, is a counter-natural (*againft nature*) Heŝtick (*deeply fix'd*) latent (*hidden*) and equal diminution, extenuation, or rather a wafting of all the parts of the body, notwithftanding the daily ingeftion (*taking*) of food with appetite. Whence appears, that the diminution or wafting of ones flefh in Feavers, is not to be termed a Confumption, becaufe that extenuation is acute, and Schetical (*fuperficial,*) that is violently quick, not lafting, and of no difficult cure; whereas in a Confumption the diminution is flow, durable, fix'd or habitual, and yeilding to no eafie cure. Neither can it be reputed a Confump-

C 3

tion,

tion, where the body is suddenly extenuated by fasting, that being rather a disease of the mind, refusing a timely supply of food to the body. Moreover it's requisite the extenuation *(wasting)* should be universal, and not of some parts only, as in a Dropsie, where the upper alone do undergo a diminution, and the lower an increase *(or swelling;)* nor of a single part, in which case it's stiled an *Atrophy*, or withering of a part; as an Atrophy of an Arm, Leg, Toe, or Finger. Lastly, the diminution of parts must be latent *(hidden,)* not caused by an over-labouring, or want of sleep, or by being over liberal in satisfying Womens impertinences, the causes whereof as they are externally obvious, so they imply no Consumption; though indeed there be a manifest shrinking of the flesh, especially in the last instance, *viz.* excess of *Amours* * (lust) which in many we may observe to cause the appearance of a perfect Consumptive, or *Hippocratical face*, as hollow Eyes, a sharp Nose, shrunk Visage, &c. Insomuch that it's impossible to distinguish them from the last degree of Consumptives, but by their

having

nereal
orts.

aving a livid circle about their Eyes, (a pe-
uliar sign of a goatish extenuation) their
chetical (*sudden*) leanness, and the absence
f an *Hectick* Feaver.

Many through their extenuation by a
ourse of Physick do oft put a fallacy upon
eoples fancies, that judge them Consump-
ve, and particularly those that are Physick
r a Clap, whose specifick (*particular*) dis-
osition of body at that time is in a fortnights
hysicking to be reduced to an *Hippocratean*
(shrunck Consumptive) Visage, in such
rt, that their acquaintance do usually give
em up for lost; but herein their state is
fferenced from a proper Consumption,
at upon their entrance into a course of
hysick, they are apt in a very short time
lose their flesh, so as to counterfeit Ana-
mies, and afterwards upon the least inter-
ission of their Medicines to impinguate
(*grow fat*) to admiration; besides their
cil (*easie*) support of churlish Remedies,
hich none but Pockifyed Patients could
stain with so small an impair of strength.

CHAP. V.

Of the nature of a Proper and True Consumption.

IN the preceeding Chapter, we have set down a description of a Consumption in general, comprehending a Proper or True, and Improper or False Consumption. Our present purpose is to begin with the first, and give you a brief, but plain, explanation thereof. Wherefore note, that Physicians when terming a Disease, (but in their sense it's rather a Symptom) a Consumption, do for the most part intend a Proper Consumption, which we do here describe, *To be an habitual* (or h ctick, confirm'd or radicated) *slow extenuation against nature ; or rather a devouring of the Fleshy and Spermatick parts of the body, through an immediate slow corruption of the Essential mixture, viz. the Radical moisture, and the Innate heat.* Whence you may deduct, that ordinary

exe-

extenuations of a Month or two, more or
lefs, are not to be nominated Proper Confumptions, which relating to the profound
Balfamick mixture fpeak great danger of
death, difficulty of cure, and implicitly a
long fpace of time before any fuch offence
againft nature can be offer'd, becaufe of the
deep latency (*hidden fituation*) of the
fubftantial principles.

Confumptive extenuations muft be *againft
nature*, to exclude natural ones, occafioned
through want of food, required to fill up the
vacuities (*empty fpaces between the Pores*)
of the parts, that happen through their daily
diffipation (*or diffolution;*) but *it's rather
an Abforbing* (fucking up) *or devouring of
the parts by Corrupting their Fundamentals*,
whereby every part doth not only fhrink,
but grows fenfibly lefs in its fubftance, fo as
the parts, as far as they are confumed, can
never be recovered, or made greater, by
reafon of the diffolution and corruption of
their *Fundamental mixture*, and the return
of their fubftantial principles into their firft
elements; unlefs it were poffible to infufe
new fubftantials into them, which to imagine
faifible,

faisible, portends a man to want a grain of
his right Reason; and certainly none but
such, as pretend to be meer Chymists, would
assert, that Potable Gold (*aurum potabile*,
or Gold Chymically reduced to a liquor, or
a thin oyle, thereby being render'd potable,
or fit to be dranck) contains a vertue of
recruiting or augmenting Natures Essentials;
which if possible, it's requisite the said *Potable Gold* should be endued with a capacity of
being agglutinated (*glewed,*) and assimilated
(*converted into a likeness*), to the *Innate
heat* and *Radical moisture*; or at least be
virtuated with a power of generating the said
essentials out of the humours within the
Vessels. The former of these instanced
ways is rejected, because it's impossible a
mineral (as Gold is) that is inanimate, (*dead*)
and incapable of receiving life, and of another *genus* (kind,) should be converted into
the highest and purest degree of an animate
substance, as the Spermatick essentials are;
for if minerals are not convertible into another *Species*, though of the same *Genus*, much
less can they be surmised reducible into a
Species of another *Genus*. Certainly what
can

can not be expected from animated plants,
yea *Animals (living moving Creatures,)*
which though belonging to the fame *Genus*
are only convertible into flefh and other
diffipable parts , but not into Spermatick
ones) it's a vanity to look far in dead minerals. Touching the vain effects of *Aurum
potabile* you may read more at large in the
fecond part of my Philofophy Book 1. *Chap.*
1. *Par.* 5. In *fumma,* unlefs it were imaginable to infufe the fame animate living Sperm
into the fubftance and penetrails *(depth)* of
the parts, it's ridiculous to expect repara-
tion from any other means ; which makes it
apparent, that it's more eafie to generate a
new man, than to repair one, that's partly
confumed in his fubftantials. This by the
way ; but to return to the explanation of the
foreftated defcription : Putrid Feavers depend upon the putrefaction *(or a tendance to
Corruption)* of the blood, whofe immediate
effect is the corruption of the faid nutritive
(nourifhing) humours , but mediately and
fwiftly (if tending to death) corrupting the
effential principles of the parts ; whereas in
a Proper Confumption the corruption is
immediate ,

immediate, and flow. Likewife other
Difeafes, as Dropfies, Jaundifes, Ptificks, *&c.*
to arrive to the period of life, muft neceffarily caufe a corruption of the effentials,
though flow, yet not immediately, but mediately by corrupting the blood.

Not to be deficient in any thing, that may
add to the illuftration of the fubject of this
Chapter, we fhall annex *Galen's* definition
of a *Simple Tabes*, or perfect Confumption;
*lib. de Tabe. A Confumption is the dying of
a living Creature through dryneſs.* This
defcription is generical, extenfible to Confumptions of Ulcerated Lungs, and thofe
that attend fimple Hectick Feavers; and fo
far it's agreeing to ours, that it confirms the
latter branch, *viz.* that it's a devouring
corruption of the effential mixture, which
confifting chiefly of an oyly moifture is cor-
ruptible through diffipation, or being dryed
away, which *Galen* here intends by *dryneſs,* to
wit the drying away of the Balfamick moifture. Moreover *Galen's* Commentators make
mention of a two fold dryneſs, the one concomitated with a heat, which they call a
Torrid Tabes; the other with a coldneſs,
termed

:rmed *Ex morbo Senium* , when the parts
:e confumed through extinction of their
ative heat, and diffipation of their *Radical*
toifture.Gal. in the forecited Book fubjects
ll the parts of the body to a fimple Con-
mption or *Tabes*, excepting the Lungs,
/hich being of a moift and foft temperature
:em not at all difpofed to fufcept any dry-
.efs. But on the contrary, it's ordinary for
miths, Cooks, and others, whofe imploy-
nent is converfant about the Fire , to
ncurre fuch an extreme drynefs of their
.ungs, that in the diffection of their Car-
affes, they appear liker Spunges than moift
.ungs; the like obfervation you'l read
)elow touching the withered Lungs of one
°endarves.

CHAP.

CHAP. VI.

Of the nature and kinds of Bastard Consumptions.

IMproper or Bastard Consumptions are only slow growing extenuations *(or wast- ings)* of the fleshy parts, directly moving to a True and Proper Consumption, by rea- son of some indisposition of the intern parts, humours, and influent spirits. In proper Consumptions there is a devouring of the Spermatick parts, and essentials, here only of the flesh and humours. So that a Bastard Consumption is curable with ease, because it's no more than a superficial and growing malady, relating to the consumed fleshy parts; but the other implyes a very diffi- cult cure, not by restoring the Spermatick parts, (which as we shewed in the preceed- ing Chapter is impossible;) but only by stenting and removing the corruption of the forementioned *essentials.*

A

A Baftard Confumption chiefly compre-
ends thefe following. 1. *An Hypochon-*
driack Confumption. 2. *A Scorbutick Con-*
fumption. 3. *An Amourous Confumption.*
4. *A Confumption of Grief.* 5. *A Studious*
Confumption. 6. *An Apoftematick Confump-*
tion. 7. *A Cancerous Confumption.* 8. *An*
Ulcerous Confumption. 9. *A Dolorous Con-*
fumption. 10. *An Aguish Confumption.*
11. *A Febril Confumption.* 12. *A Cachectick*
Confumption. 13. *A Verminous Confumption.*
14. *A Confumption of the Rickets.* 15. *A*
Pockie Confumption. 16. *A Poyfonous Con-*
fumption. 17. *A Bewitch'd Confumption.*
18. *A Confumption of the Back.* 19. *A*
Confumption of the Kidneys. 20. *A Con-*
fumption of the Lungs.

All thefe tending to a True Confumption,
unlefs anticipated *(prevented)* by a mortal
acute Difeafe, do juftly come under the notion of Baftard, or growing Confumptions.
Neither is't our purpofe to treat farther of
of thefe Difeafes, than relating to Confumptions, the manner whereof, how they may be
conceived to caufe fuch extenuations, we
fhall fuccinctly *(in fhort)* fet down in
particular Chapt. CHAP.

CHAP. VII.

Of an Hypochondriack Consumption.

AN Hypochondriack Consumption is an
extenuation of the fleshy parts, occasioned by an infarction (*clogging and over
filling,*) and obstruction of the Spleen,
pancreas, mesaraick, and Stomachick Veffels, through melancholly, or grofs, dreggish,
tartarous humours; whereby it happeneth,
the blood is not fufficiently defæcated, or
clarifyed, but remains muddy, and ditchy,
which stagnating (*standing still without motion*) thus for a while turns saltish and
acrimonious, offending and perverting the
Stomach, Spleen, and Liver in their Offices,
a neceffary precedent of vitiated (*foul*)
blood, which being rejected by the parts,
the body muft needs fall away for want of
better nutriture (*nourifhment.*) This salin
fap of the Veffels for being refufed recep-
tion of the parts, indues daily a greater
ferocity

rocity *(fierceness,)* and declares it self in more hostile *(like an Enemy)* manner, insinuating *(peircing)* into the profundi- *(depth)* of the parts, and so drying, sorbing *(sucking up,)* and consuming the *adical moisture* and *Innate heat,* arrives to Proper Consumption. Add hereunto the ntinual vigilies *(overwaking,* or *want of ep,)* melancholique, sorry, dull, lingring flions, the said Hypochondriack patient præcipitated *(forced)* into, whereby the irits being rendred dull, stupid, languid *ainting),*and suppressed, are deserted *(left)* capable of ventilating *(breathing)* and irifying the blood, and debilitated *(weaked)* in attracting *(drawing)* nutriment r the parts, which consequently must ither and shrink. It's no wonder there- re so many Melancholicks do daily drop to perfect Consumptions, since their præous *(foregoing)* indisposition doth so diⅇtly tend to an absolute marcour *(dry-fs.*

Among the rest of the Entrails, we have iserted the Spleen the chief seat of this *Hypochondriack* evil,against which assertion
D m'ay

may be objected ; that the Spleen rather seems to be superadded for some use, than any publick function of defæcating (*clari- fying,*) or engendring blood. The use allotted for it, may be to fill up that empty space, that would be, if the Spleen were wanting, or to transmit heat to the Stomach for to promote digestion, or to serve for a supporter to the Veins and Arteries, that pass through it to several parts of the body. That its not destined for any absolute neces- sary function of generating or clarifying the blood, is inferred from that ancient custome, *Plautus, Haliabbas* and *Pliny* lib.11.cap.37. speak of, where they were wont to burn the Spleen of their foot coursers, that used to run for sport or wagers, and some they would quite cut out their Spleen, to make them run lighter, and render them long winded ; be- cause the Spleen is otherwise apt to weigh down the *Diaphragma* (Midriff,) which is a chief instrument of Respiration. *Ron- sæus* in his Treatise de *Part. Cas. Sect.* 4, *cap.* 5. inserts an observation of several, whose Spleen were cut out ; and of another, whose Spleen was quite worn or dryed

away,

ray, and nothing remaining but the out-
ird skin. We do eafily admit of the poffi-
lity of the forefaid practice, fince I have
en a tryal made of it upon a Dog, but with
is confequence, that it certainly fhortens
e, and renders the remaining courfe im-
exed with fundry troubles and difeafes. In
e mean time that office, which we allow
e Spleen, is performed by the Liver,
increas, and other parts, though with fome
fficulty, becaufe they are overtask'd; for
ubtlefs in that cafe the groffer part of the
ood is evacuated by the *Hæmorrhoids*, as
s ufual in other accidents, when the body
mutilated *(deprived)* of an Arm or Leg.
that it appears, the Office of the Spleen
of great importance, though it may be
plyed by other parts in cafe it be difeafed,
ftructed, or exected *(cut out.)* The fame
ception might be ftarted againft the Liver;
r were it not for the effufion of blood of
ofe great veins, that have their root in it,
r according to others terminate there,)
hich would neceffarily follow an exection,
e Liver might not only be exected, but
's Office likewife fupplyed by the Spleen

and

and the other parts.   Since I have drawn
my Reader a little out of the way by this
objection, I shall conduct him back to the
remainder of this Chapter, which is a brief
inventory of the Signs of an *Hypochondriack*
Consumption, that so he may not be sur-
prized with the fate of it. 1. There is a
frequent rumbling noise under the Stomach,
thwarting from the right side to the left, and
thence back again. 2 Pinching pains about the
Stomach, as if they would girt a mans body
close together. 3. Glowing heats under the
short Ribs. 4. Frequent belchings, that
smell sowre, or stink. 5. A windiness and
puffing up of their Stomach, especially after
dinner, and in the morning after they wake.
6. Much spitting.   7. Vomiting, or at least
an inclination to Vomit. 8. If upon these
Signs you find a wasting of your flesh, than
look about you, especially if troubled with
a Cough.

CHAP.

CHAP. VIII.

Of a Scorbutick Consumption.

THe Scurvy is diſcovered a Melancholique Diſeaſe through its dreggiſh tartarous Eruptions, as courſe boils, puſtles, *&c.*
wherein it's differenced from *Hypochondriack melancholy*, whoſe *tartar* (melancholy) is retained within the body, & for that
reaſon proves by far more incommodious (as
appears by thoſe doleful paſſions,) which if
it were propelled (*caſt forth*,) in Boils, Bot-
ches, or Ulcers, as in the Scurvy, would
rather conduce to health, thoſe ſharp ſcorbu-
tick dregs imitating the nature of yiſt, in
cauſing the blood to ferment or work out into thoſe eruptions (*breakings out*,) whereby
the blood is wonderfully clarifyed and purged. Hence it is, that many Melancholiques
and Splenetick perſons are of an exceeding
merry and cheerful diſpoſition ; by reaſon
their melancholy by cauſing their blood to

D 3 work

work, doth so much clarify it, whereout the spirits must needs afterwards be generated very clear, lucid, (*light*) and lively.

But of this I have discoursed more at large in *Venus unmask'd, Book. 1. Art.* 37. *Par.* 134, 135. however though the Scurvy proves so healthful during its commence-ment (*beginning*) and augment (*increase,*) yet being once advanced to a state, is found to have indued a more disobliging and cor-roding nature, (as appears by those arthritick (*gowty*) night pains, and Phagedenick (*raw*) Ulcers it causes : Read my *Vener. Discovery Book.* 1. *Art.* 9. *Par.* 39.) through the per-mutation (*change*) of its *Nitrous* and *Vi-triolat salt* into an *Armoniack*, which par-taking of so penetrating and corrosive a na-ture, doth soon attaque the fleshy, and immediately after make towards the cor-rupting of the Fundamental parts.

A Scorbutick Consumption is easily dis-cerned by observing a lingring wasting of ones flesh upon a prævious (*foregoing*) Scurvy, attended with a Cough; the Signs of a Scurvy I have set down in *Venus Unmask'd.*

CHAP.

CHAP. IX.

Of an Amorous Consumption.

OF all Baſtard Conſumptions none doth more rapidly (*ſwiftly*) occaſion an ꜩtenuation of the fleſh, than an Amorous ꜩondition, which where it doth faſten, im‑ꜩediately cauſes a very ſenſible falling of ꜩe countenance; whence it's a common ꜩjeċtion, when Maids do ſuddenly grow ꜩn‑jawed and hallow‑eyed, they are cer‑ꜩinly in Love. Neither is there cauſe want‑ꜩg for ſo ſubitous (*ſudden*) an alteration, ꜩhere there is ſuch a lingring, ſighthing, ꜩbbing, and looking after the return of the ꜩſent objeċt, the thoughts ſo fix'd, that they ꜩe imployed upon nothing but the paſt ꜩſion; & the mind all that while ſo diſturbed ꜩd perplex'd with hopes, doubts, fears, ꜩſſibilities, and improbabilities, that the ꜩart ſtrikes five hundred ſorts of Pulſes in an ꜩur; and hunted into ſuch continual palpi‑

D 4　　　　　　tations

tations through anxiety (*oppreſſion*) and diſtraction, that (as the ſaying is) fain would it break if it could. By means of all which alterations, violent motions, frights, fears, and other paſſions, the Animal (*ſpirits of the brain*) and Vital (*of the heart*) ſpirits ſuffer ſuch loſſes and diſperſions, that we ſee its ordinary for young Wenches to be reduced to faintings, ſownings, and extreme weakneſſes, to the admiration of their parents, whence ſuch ſubitous and effrayable (*frightful*) ſymptoms ſhould ſource (*take their riſe.*) *Galen* among the reſt of his remarques (*lib. de pracogn. ad Poſthum. cap. 6.*) tells us of a *Woman* patient of his, whom he found very weak in bed, continually toſſing and tumbling from one ſide to the other, and totally deprived of her reſt. No extern or intern cauſe could he diſcover of this malady, neither would ſhe contribute any thing of her own confeſſion, though he oft required it of her, which kind of mute (*dumb*) deportment gave him ſuſpicion of ſome melancholy, or love buſineſs the woman was troubled with; however he repeated his viſits the ſecond and third time, though

ough with as little satisfaction as before; ut at last it happened one came to visit her, nd told her she had been at the Theater, here she had seen *Pylades* (one of the layers) dance, whereupon *Galen* observed er to change her countenance, and immeiately feeling her pulse, found it to beat ery various and disturbed, a sign of some rouble of the mind, and so perceiving the ame disturbance of her pulse, as oft as *Pylades* was discoursed of, was confirm'd in is opinion, that all those symptoms were a roduct (*effect*) of her *love*. *Aretaus lib.* 3. *ap.* 3. instances likewise a young man, nvolved in the same passion, and surprized with the worst of symptoms. And beyond ll this *Valer. Max. lib.* 5. *cap.* 7. records *Antiochus* the only Son of the King *Seleucus*, deeply fallen in love with *Stratonica* his Mother-in-law, who piously dissembling his burning passion, præcipitated himself into a most dangerous Consumption, the cause whereof his Physitian *Erasistratus* could in no-ways descry, before such time as *Stratonica* entring the room, moved a blushy colour in his face, and rendred his aspect

vivacious

vivacious (*lively*,) but deserting him, he soon relapsed to the same paleness and languor (*faintness*;) which ebbing and flowing of his countenance with the uncertainty of his pulse, certifyed *Erasistratus*, of some love wound his Mother had struck upon his heart; and declaring this accident to the King his Father, almost cast down with grief for his Son, now ee'n strucken with his last fate, he soon yeilded his dearest wife for a remedy to *Antiochus*, considering it was chance, striving with his unparallel'd modesty and bashfulness, had reduced him to that extremity. *Hippocrates* shewed himself no less skilful in discerning the discriminous (*dangerous*) state of *Perdiccas* King of *Macedonia*, occasioned by the doting love he harbour'd in his breast for *Phila*, one of his Fathers Concubines, whose presence at any time excited a great alteration of his pulse. But these passages that resent so much of natures impressions, do in no wise merit to be admired at, when brutish dotings prove so efficacious in impelling bodies into a marcour (*extreme leanness*;) as Historians verifie of a rich *Athenian*, and indifferently

rently

ently defcended, who fpying a marble
Statue erected in a publick place of *Athens,*
and very curioufly wrought, grew fo paffio-
nate upon it, that he fpent whole nights in
imbracing it, at laft defirous to impropriate
this object to himfelf, wooed the Senat
to part with it, offering to lay down a
treble value ; but they cenfuring it impious,
to make Merchandize of what belonged to
the publick, denyed his importune requeft,
whereupon he increafed in fondnefs, and
beftowed a Golden Crown upon it, Cloath-
ing it alfo with rich and coftly Apparel,
adored, and oft proftrated himfelf before
it, which the Senat judging indecent, forbad
him making any more addreffes to their
Statue. The young *Athenian* finding himfelf deprived of his joy and delight, fell into
a Confumption, and before that could limit
the courfe of his life, he cut his own throat.
This paffion was not fo ridiculous, but it
was exceeded by the King *Xerxes*, whom
many Authours affirm to have been ftrangely
inamoured upon an Oak, which he would
oft hug and kifs, as if it had been fome pretty Woman. Many more modern inftances
we

we could produce to illustrate the force of
this sort of passion upon bodies, which we
refer to another place. These commotions
of the mind and body do after a short continuance menace (*threaten*) a Consumption,
by oppressing the heart and its vital spirits
with such throngs of blood and spirits, that
are impelled and propt into its Ventricles,
(*small hollow rooms within the heart*)whereby
the heart is choak'd and obstructed in its
pulsation (*beating,*) and consequently hin-
dred from transmitting vital blood to the
parts, which for want thereof must necessarily wither and dry away ; moreover in that
case the blood grows thick and muddy for
want of motion, and so acquires an ill quality, and causes obstructions , as we have
expressed in the preceding Chapter ; besides
the spirits growing dull and stupid do not
perform their office in drawing the blood to
the several parts, which must necessarily add
very much to the wasting of the body. Lastly,
if those love frights prove very violent, the
blood and spirits returning in great streams
to the heart, may not only suddenly choak
it, but also extinguish its Innate spirits, and

o that doting paſſion happens to terminate (end) into a mortal *Syncope* (ſwoun;) thus *Euryalus* a Knight belonging to the Empeour *Sigiſmund,* taking leave of his Miſtriſs *Lucretia* of *Siena*, præcipitated her into ſuch a Love fit, that within a few hours after ſhe Ghoſted; which courſe *Euryalus* was like to have ſteered, upon the news of that ſad accident, had his paſſion not been diverted, by ſome recreation his friends gave him. The like fate befell a *Dutch* Gentlewoman, upon the ſudden death of her Puppy dog, which ſhe doted upon beyond imagination, as the Scene afterwards atteſted.

But young bloſſom'd Girls ſeem to be troubled with another Divil within 'em, to augment *(increaſe)* the fire of their doting hell, and that's their *Mother,* which muſt ever and anon be a fuming up to their throats upon the leaſt diſturbance of their *Amours* (love,) as I have oft been a Spectator of ſeveral, that fell into moſt terrible fits of the Mother, five or ſix in a day, upon a rupture of Marriage. I ſhall finiſh this Chapter with a ſhort obſervation of the Prognoſticks *(foreſayings)* of this *Amorous* Conſumption,

tion. Young wenches once thoroughly smitten with Love darts, seldome or never lose that first impression, though they may be diverted by their parents, in shewing them an imparity (*unsutablenefs*) in their Fortunes, Families, Perfons, &c. and therefore must be compelled to marry such others, as their Parents pleafe, perhaps being perfwaded by fome Bawdy-Broaker, who (according to the ancient cuftome) takes ten in the hundred for fo much portion he Procures, and fo much Joynture anfwerable to the current rate of the market, much after the form Cows are fold in *Smithfield*, according to the goodnefs of their Hides and Tallow. In the mean while thefe poor Laffes droop away, between a lingring after their firft Loves, and a certain chaftity that forbids 'em eating Fifh and Flefh in one day. The only prevention of this great mifchief is, to imitate the Jewifh cuftome, to pen up their Daughters, and let them be acquainted with none, but fuch as they certainly intend for their Husbands; for beyond contradiction their firft Love ftands againft all oppofition of imparities of fortunes,

families,

families, or any thing whatfoever, as this
narrative witneffes of a Princefs of *France*,
who walking melancholique alone in the
field, fell in difcourfe with a *Flemifh* Shepherds, and finding his perfon, talk, gefture,
and tone of fpeech quite different from the
Court Company, began to admire him,
and grew fo much enamour'd upon him, that
before their parting, they defign'd their fe-
cret tranfportation into *Flanders* ; to which
purpofe fhe put her felf into the Garb of a
Shepherdefs, and in that difguife lived many
years ; but difcovering her felf a little before
her death, did profefs her felf the happieft
perfon alive, not for her condition, but in
injoying him fhe firft loved, and that fhe
would rather ten Thoufand times choofe to
live a Shepherdefs (notwithftanding the hardnefs and vilenefs that attend fo defpicable a
life) in the contentment and fatisfaction of
her Shepherd, than the glorious life of a
Princefs. If upon this you require a cenfure,
I can but fay, it was the humour of a Woman. Neither do I find men lefs eftranged
to extravagancies in this particular ; *Lucius
Vitellius*, the Father of *Vitellius* the *Roman*
Emperour,

Emperour, a Sage and Prudent person,
was so affectionately taken with a common
Strumpet, that he would never suffer her to
spit on the ground, but alwayes saved her
spittle in a golden Vessel he carried about
with him for the same purpose, whereunto
he added so much Honey as would make it
into a Syrup, which he was wont to lick with
the greatest delight imaginable. This relation doth not so much savour of folly, as that
of *Galeazo* (Duke of *Mantua*) of madness, he whilst sojourning at *Padua* had so
enslaved himself to a fond passion upon a
Wench, that upon her commanding him to
drown himself, he immediately gave Spur
to his Horse, and so plunged himself head-
long into the River. The great *Charlemain*,
who was master of the better part of *Europe*,
yet could not Master the passion he bore to a
Gentlewoman, whom after she was dead,
he would not suffer to be removed out of
his Bed-Chamber in order to her Funeral,
and though she stunk like a Carrion, yet
sented to him like a Violet. What treachery
men harbour within their breast to betray
'em to their greatest Enemy, Death! what a
strange

range inchantment, that renders men thus
wilfully fottifh, melancholique, mad, and
defperate! Certainly this muft be fome kind
of curfe intailed upon mankind, for having
originally groffely tranfgreffed in that particular. But what remedy to refift fo great
an evil? Women in this cafe require the
precedency of cure, as being the firft occafion of that fin, and firft caufe of the curfe,
witnefs elfe their mother *Eve*, who could
fhe but have paffed by that finful curiofity,
God Almighty in his wifdome had referved
more noble way of man's propagation, in
lieu, that whereas man is now begotten in the
burning Sin of luft like a beaft, and born
creeping out of his mothers belly downwards towards the earth with fhame, he
would have been begotten in a more fpiri-
tual manner, and have been born glorioufly,
making his firft afcenfion towards the heavens to falute his Creator. But to our dooms
we do ftill find the daughters of *Eve* perfift-
ing in their mothers curiofity, in alluring the
poor Sons of *Adam* to all manner of lafci-
vioufnefs and debauchery; and to that purpofe they plaifter their faces with patches,

E   rub

rub their skin with white Lead, and go naked to the very Paps (and they are like they say in *France*, to fall into the Amazones mode of waring short coats to reach no farther than their knees;) and in this posture will they be leaning out of their Balcones and Windows, frisking and gigling, that they would e'en tempt a Saint;

Ten teems of Oxen draw much less
Than one hair of a Womans tress.

But all this is but speculation or dumb leche-ry; the practick part consists in their goatish discourses, winking at Church, going to Dancing-Schools, Plays, Spring-Gardens, Taverns, and where not.

Kissing though repeated hundred times over, is a piece of their Dancing-School breeding, that's not to be refused; and what saith the *Italian* to this, *Donna basciata mezzo guadagnata*, a *woman* kissed is half conquer'd. How these creatures may be reformed, has been the study of many ages, though as we see to little purpose.

Thus far they all agree, women ought
to

keep within and seldome stir out; and
en they go forth, the *Italians* will have
m to have neither eyes nor ears; that is,
y must not stair men in the face like
cks, nor listen after idle talk. Neither
they think it necessary for 'em to go to
urch, imagining a Woman doth very well
rit her salvation, in doing penance of
eping her self honest at home; besides, in
itation of *Ovid's* dictate, *Otia si tollas
iere cupidinis arcus*, they would have them
ployed twenty hours a day in Spinning,
itting, *&c.* the rest of the time in
ting and sleeping.

In short, these three Devises are necessary
make an honest Woman; Retiredness,
eligion, and Employment. On the con-
ary, where a Woman is used to Company,
d little regards Religion, and is less im-
loyed, there's you know what.

However, notwithstanding all these diver-
sements, they will now and then take an
ccasion to fall in Love, though it be but by
ear-say, as *Guyon* writes in his *divers Lecons
. part fol.* 365. of three Gentlewomen,
at fell strangely in love with one and the

E 2   same

same person. The Story runs thus: It happened that a Waiting-Gentlewoman to the Dutchess of *Urbin*, took a great liking to a Gentleman, belonging to the same Court; but her modesty being such, as would not suffer her to declare her affection immediately to him, advised with another Gentlewoman a friend of hers about it, to whom she opened her breast, expressing likewise the merits and personage of the Gentleman; whose Characters agreeing so well with her own Phantie, she (namely the second Gentlewoman) grew furiously inamour'd upon the party described, and thereupon in stead of solliciting for her friend, she put Pen to Paper and wrote a most passionate Letter for her self, and addressed it to the foresaid Gentleman; this letter fell accidently into the hands of a third Gentlewoman, who upon the reading thereof was inflamed in Love to the same person, beyond any of the others, and began to push hard for herself: But fortune proved so just to them all, that because of their rash indiscreet passions, they lost their pains, and went all without him. *Valent. Bruchius* a *Spaniard* relates a passage

not

not unlike this, of a Dutchefs of *Savoy*, who fell defperately in Love with a Knight of the Family of *Mendoza*, only by hearing his Sifter fay, *Would to God this Princefs were Married to my Brother, and they would make the moft glorious couple in the world, for perfection and beauty.* This fucceeded fo happily, that fome time after (as the common faying is) they had one another. Thefe two Narratives afford us another moral to be added as a fourth to the three forementioned deviles, to wit a young Maid muft not only be kept in a perpetual retirement, devotion, and conftant imployment, but muft not fo much as be entertained with a difcourfe of love, or young men, for fear of raifing that evil fpirit, which afterwards would not be eafily allayed.

Now, though a fole rectification of Womens corrupt paffions (they by their allurements, gefticulations (*wanton actions*) fleering looks, and lafcivious difcourfes, being the prime movents, and inciters of this curfed inclination) were a means efficacious enough to prevent mens fottifh affections, yet we will appofe an inftance or two,

E 3 whereby

whereby you may obferve how eafily men are checked in their amorous appetites.

Raimundus Lullius, a great proficient in Chymical Philofophy, chanced to be furioufly taken with the beauty of a certain young Woman, and being impatient of his Love flames, did vehemently importune her to allay his paffion; whereupon fhe prefixt a day, which *Raimund* in no wife forgot to pafs by, but prefented himfelf at the very moment: The fair Lady, like a Goddefs of chaftity, in ftead of gratifying his beaftly luft, fuddenly flung open her bofome, and offer'd a moft filthy, ftinking, ulcer'd Cancer of her Breaft to his view, in defign to relax, or rather break the ftrings of his Satyrick paffion, which took fo good an effect, that *Raimund* now bore greater refpects to her for her chaftity, than ever he did for her beauty. But becaufe a fole example is fo fcant an illuftration, I fhall not think it much to contribute another no lefs remarkable than the former. *Hypatia* the Phenix of her time, both for her incomparable wit, and excellent beauty, had the fortune of being moft fondly doated upon by a young Scholar,

cholar; the force of whose inclinations
was so puissant (*strong,*) that it was like to
npell him into a distraction : the unparallel
hastity of this virtuous Female could in no
ind be prevailed with to favour him in what
e so passionately aimed at, though her com-
assion, sensible of the torment he endured
n that amourous hell, would have com-
lyed in whatever had been consistent with
ne nature of modesty. At length she disco-
ered to her self an ingenious cure, to reme-
y the poor Schollar of his menaced insany
madness,) in order whereunto, knowing
im to be master of a great deal of reason,
ne muster'd a great bundle of her menstru-
us rags together (as the wise man calls
nem, and spread them all open before
im ; saying, you men that do so admire at
ne Elegant shape, and Nitourous Com-
exion of Womens upper parts, behold
ow, O Scholar ! the constitution of their
ower, the object of all your Lascivious
oves; what a filthy, nasty, detestable sight
here ? whereat the ingenuous Scholar took
ch a regret, having been hitherto deluded,
crediting this dictate of *Hermes, Quod*

E 4   *est*

eſt ſuperius, eſt ſicut inferius. That is, whatever is above is like to what is below ; that ever after he abhorred the ſight of a Woman. If arguments of this kind, drawn from the falſe appearance of Women , would take with the generality of men, there's enough to be ſaid to fling 'em all out of favour. But enough of this.

CHAP. IX.

Of a Conſumption of Grief.

GRief protracted to ſome ſpace of time, doth inevitably *(unavoidably)* abſorb *(ſuck up)* the fleſhy parts of the body, and ſtrait-way haſten to a perfect Conſumption. Grief is a pain of the ſoul for the abſence of ſome good thing, or the preſence of an evil thing.   Now, as far as the ſoul o'retops the body, ſo far its pains , or rather mournful ſenſations, exceed thoſe of the Carcaſſe ; A Gowt, a Colick, the cutting off of an Arm or Leg, or ſearing the Fleſh with an hot

Iron,

Iron, are but Fleabits to the grieving pains of the Soul; for the being only chearful, doth as eafily conquer, as endure them. But it's otherwife with the body, that immediately fhrinks under the leaft pain of the Soul.

Among the varieties of Grief, the controverfie of the greateft, is folely depending between *Grief* taken for a *difgrace*, and *Grief* for the lofs of a *Relation :* And both thefe are fuch, as will attaque (*fall upon*) and conquer the wifeft and moft couragious of either Sex ; Reafon in either of thefe cafes can produce no other, than trifling arguments to fupprefs 'em. All ranks of Nobles and Ignobles are obferved, to yeeld to the fury of thefe Soul-pains. *Bajazed* the *Turkifh* Emperour, and *Tamerlan*'s Prifoner, rather than to fuftain the difgrace of being carried about in an Iron cage, chofe death, by running his head againft the Grates.

Senca's Wife prefer'd dying with her Husband, before fhe would furvive to grieve for his death.

Cecinna Petus being fentenced to death, but with a refervation, that he might make choice

choice of his own way of dying, *Arrion* his Wife came to him, though full of grief, and in his sight drew a Dagger, and stabbed her self, crying out, the wound I have made doth not pain me, but the wound that thou wilt make, O *Pete!* pains me.

To give you an Emblem of a more Chronical (*of a longer time*) operation of grief, wee'l commend a Narrative or two more to your Reading.

One Captain *Munck* a Dane, famous for the Expedition he performed to the North, to discover a nearer passage to the *Indies*, after a most dangerous Winter-quarter returned home, to give an account of his Voyage to the King of *Danemark* his Master; who being dis-satisfied at his deportment, thrusted the said Captain from him with his Cane, whereupon he took his leave, and went home, but with such a resentment of the disgrace, that some few dayes after he put forward to another world.

The like Scene we observe in *Don Olivares* the great Favourite of *Spain*, who soon rendred his life to the conquest of grief he took

for

or the difgrace of being depofed of all his Offices and Dignities.

Fates not much differing from this befell alfo Cardinal *Woolfey*, and many other Grandees, upon the like occafions.

In fine, it's a common obfervation among the *Spanifh* Polititians, that the fureft Stratagem, to be quite rid of a Statefman, that ftands in the way, and befides to avoid popular clamours and cenfures, is to depofe him of all his dignities, and imprifon him, where without queftion the apprehenfion of his difgrace, or the pernicious air of a Prifon, will foon fet a period to the courfe of his days, or at leaft put him upon fome revengeful attempt, whereby he may be rendred a riper objeʃt for a publick Scene.

This by the way, to illuftrate to you the danger of a pain in the Soul, and the near fympathy there is between her and the body.

Touching the manner of caufality, whereby grief effects fuch fierce fymptoms, *viz.* a fudden Death, and a lingring Confumption, may be collected out of the preceding difcourfe upon an Amorous Confumption, to wit, the former is caufed, through a full and

fudden

sudden irruption (*breaking in*) of thick Melancholique blood into the Ventricles (*narrow rooms*) of the heart, thereby choaking
the vital spirits, and putting a stop to the
hearts pulsation, which if intermitted but
three or four Pulses, portends a certain death.
The latter is atchieved by a gradual suppression of the vital spirits, through heavy
tartarous (*dreggish*)blood, which (namely the
spirits) defecting, must necessarily cause an
extinction of the innate heat and spirits, for
whose nutrition they are designed, and so consequently a perfect Consumption must be the
ultimate issue. Add hereto the restlesness
and intermission from sleep grieved persons are molested with, whereby the blood
is much dryed, the spirits consumed, and
melancholy increased.

Moreover, as melancholick blood doth so
much suppress the vital spirits, so it's very
unapt for ministring matter for new spirits,
or being converted into flesh, because of its
grossenes and crudity. Neither doth that
blood continue long so, as I said before, but
acquires an acrimony, whereby it's much
intended (*heightned*) in its devouring and
consuming quality.   CHAP.

CHAP. X.

Of a Studious Consumption.

MOderate labour of the body is univerfally experienced to conduce to the
prefervation of health, and curing many
initial (*beginning*) Difeafes; but on the
contrary, the toyle of the mind, to deftroy
health and generate Maladies, by attracting
the fpirits out of the entire body from their
task of Concoction, Diftribution, and Excretion, to the brain, whither they carry along
with them clouds of vapours and excrementitious humours of the whole, thereby excef-
fively annoying the brain and its faculties,
impelling it into various Difeafes, as *Catarrhs*, (*defluxions of humours*,) ftupors,
(*numnefs*,) imminution (*leffening*) of the
memory and imagination; impairs of the
external fenfes, as dulnefs of hearing or
feeing, imbecillity (*weaknefs*) in ftirring
or walking, &c. Likewife the other parts of
the

the body, being deprived of their spirits, sustain very considerable damages ; as, the Stomach happeneth to be weakned in its *Concoction* , whence crudities and loss of appetit; the Spleen and Liver in their Offices of defæcation, whence vitious, melancholick, dreggish, sulphurous blood, and obstructions of the Bowels and Vessels ; the Heart in its distributing the blood to all the parts of the body, and strength of pulsation, whence an *Atrophia*, or want of nutriment in the parts, the immediate cause of a *Studious Bastard Consumption*. Add hereto a sedentary (*sitting*) life, appropriate to all Students, crushing the bowels , and for want of stirring the body, suffers the spirits to lye dormant and dull, whence costiveness, dispersing malign, putrid fumes out of the Guts and Mesentery (*a thick double skin that tyes the Guts together*) into all parts of the body, occasioning head-ach , flushing of the blood to the head, feavers, loss of appetit, and disturbance of Concoction.

It is beyond imagination to conceive the sudden destructive effects of a Studious life; some eight or ten years since there dyed at
Abington

bington one *Pendarves* , an incompara-
le hard Student, and Minilter of that Town,
ho being diffected, his Lungs were found
) be withered and dryed up into an exact
efemblance of an ordinary Spunge in point
f fubftance and bignefs.

The like Emblems we find frequently in
Iniverfities, where Scholars daily drop
way of Confumptions.

Neither is it an extraordinary obfervation,
o fee Confumptions in the Faces of hun-
lreds of the late Preaching Divines; witnefs
ilfe their thin Jaws and number of Caps.

CHAP. XI.

Of an Apoftematick Confumption.

A *Poftems*, although internal, do rarely
caufe Confumptions before they break,
unlefs feated amongft the Glandules in the
Mefentery, where I have obferved them to
occafion a very difcernable extenuation;
which Symptom feems very ftrange in that

cafe ,

cafe, fince a Phyfician can fcarce find any
fenfible caufe of fo vifible an evil, the principal intrails giving no fign of the leaft
diftemper, and the appetit confifting as for-
merly. In fuch a cafe many would impute
the forefaid Confumption to obftructions,
no other caufe, difeafe, or part appearing
fufpicious; for a deep latent *Apoftem* in
the Mefentery if of no great mole *(bignefs,)*
cannot be fenfibly difcovered, but by conjecture only; fince the touch cannot penetrate fo deep as to reach it, becaufe of its
deep fituation, neither can the relation be
expected from the Patient, becaufe the part
affected is infenfible.

In the Hofpital at *Leiden* fome twelve or
fourteen years ago, I obferved the like
accident in a boy, who perceiving his flefh
to fhrink every day more and more, although
without the leaft fenfe of any difeafe that
fhould caufe it, applyed himfelf to a Phyfician of the Town, where he then lived,
who imputed the caufe of his Confumption
to obftructions of the Liver and Spleen,
(a trodden Sanctuary for hidden difeafes,) and
prefcribed him a Deoppilative *(opening)*
and

nd Purgative *Apozem*, not queftioning his
ure. The youth finding no benefit, doubt-
d his Doctor had miftaken the Difeale ;
pon this refolves to go to the Univerfity to
ee what the Profeffors could make of it, who
ll cryed out againft Hypochondriack Obftructions, except *Prof. Lindanus*, who
conjectured it might be fome hidden abfcefs
n the *Mefentery*, which breaking fome
few days after was difcovered to be an
Apoftem of the Mefentery, by the evacuation of the matter by ftool.

How an Apoftem in the *Mefentery* breaking, caufes a Confumption of the parts, is
apparent, *viz.* by immitting purulent fumes
into the Arteries, and Veins, corrupting
and affecting the blood with a malign quality, which proving very offenfive to the
parts, in fubverting and poyfoning their
innate temperature, is rejected by 'em,
whereby they are forced to wither for want
of nutriment. The faid purulent vapours
crowding into the fubftances of the principal and fub-principal parts, *viz.* the Heart,
Brain, Spleen, and Liver, do likewife fo
infect, poifon, and deftroy their *Innate*

F tem-

temperaments , that they immediately begin to languish in their offices , to the great prejudice of all the body. But it's not so manifest by what means an *Apostem* in the *Mesentery* should occasion a *Consump-tion* before its *maturation* , or breaking, since no *purulent* fumes can be supposed to be transmitted throughout the body before a maturation , nor after, unless the humour break, because the said fumes cannot transude (*sweat*) through the bag of an Imposthum.

In my opinion the parts happen to be consumed for want of nourishment , that's intercepted from them through the Apo-stems tumid compression and coarctation of the *Mesaraick* and *Lacteal* (milky) veins, whereby the transmission of *Chyle* (*a white juice all our Victuals is turn'd into in the Stomach*) and blood is obstructed.

CHAP

CHAP. XI.

Of a Scirrous Confumption.

IT's requifite I fhould firft tell you, what a *Scirrus* is, namely a hard tumour without pain, feeling to the touch like a ftone, caufed through a concretion of melancholick extravafate (*fhed out of the veins or arteries*) Blood. Setting afide the enumeration of compound *Scirrous* tumors, viz. *Scirrous* and *Oedematique, Scirrous* and *Phlegmonique, Scirrous* and *Eryfipelous*, I fhall only infert the kinds of generation of a fimple *Scirrus*; either it's primarly generated out of the effufion of melancholick blood, or fecundarily out of the dregs and remainder of a Phlegmonous or Oedematick tumour. Either of thefe befalling the *Liver, Spleen, Stomach, Mefentery*, or any other important entrail, may caufe an extenuation of the Flefh, by compreffing the vital and nutritive Channals, and fo intercepting the courfe of the blood and vital fpirits in

F 2 their

their afflux *(flowing to)* to the parts. 2. By
vitiating *(altering to worfe)* the fubftance
and temperament of the faid Entrails,
whereby the blood is not juftly prepared for
nourifhing of the parts.

CHAP. XII.

Of a Cancerous Confumption.

Ancers invading any internal part of
the body do in fome fpace of time
through an *Arfenical Sulphur* and *Armoniack Salt(Ven.* read *unmaskt,* fol. 65 .& 67.)
their conftituent caufes , corrode the flefh,
and foon after corrupt the *Effential mixture*, which done renders them abfolutely
incurable, unlefs extirpated *(rooted out)* by
exection or amputation *(cutting off;)* which
within the body takes no place.

Hereupon the blood is foon vitiated with
a malign quality, and its Courfe obftructed,
which proves the immediate caufe of an
improper Confumption.

CHAP

CHAP. XIII.

Of an Ulcerous Confumption.

T's needlefs to premit the defcription of an Ulcer, fince its generally known ; I fhall only obferve their difference ; fome to be external, others internal ; and fome to depend upon the intemperament of the part Ulcerated, others upon the continual flux of lacerative *(taring)* humours ; and laftly, fome to be irrigated *(moiftned)* with a more malign *pus (matter,)* than others. Of thefe its certain both extern and intern to oft caufe a gradual maceration *(wafting)* of the Flefh ; but of externals only fuch, whofe *pus (matter)* is virulent *(venomous* and malign, the fteems whereof regurgiting *(flowing back)* into the Veffels, do fenfibly infect the blood and the temperament of the chief intern members, where the parts happen to be extenuated in fuch manner, as we have once or twice illuftra-

E 3 ted

ted to you already. 2. Extern Ulcers depending upon the transmission of vitiate *(foul)* humours out from within the body, do occasion an extenuation of the parts, by attracting and depriving them of their nutriment, as I once observed in a youth in the *Charitè* Hospital at *Paris*, who through the daily and copious efflux *(evacuation)* of matter through the Orifice *(mouth)* of a deep Ulcer in his Thigh, was reduced to a Skeleton, *(skin and bones,)* and so within a while after dyed of a perfect Consumption.

Intern Ulcers impell the parts into Consumptions through their purulent fumes, thereby poysoning and infecting the blood that should nourish them.

CHAP

CHAP. XIV.

Of a Dolorous Consumption.

Violent pains are only apt to caufe infla-mations and acute Feavers, which terminating to a good or evil *Crifis*, are not likely to occafion Confumptions ; fo that it's only lingring, foft, durable pains, do dif-pofe patients to them, by oft attracting the fpirits from other parts, and fpending them ; for nothing doth waft the fpirits fwifter than pains ; fo that pains for fpending of the fpi-rits of all other accidents comes neareft to the copious and fwift lofs of fpirits by *Phle-botomy (opening of a Vein :)* Now how the diminution of fpirits caufes a Confumption we have fet down before in the preceding Chapters.

Add hereto the interception of fleep that pains occafion , which doth very much in-creafe the difperfing and depopulating of the faid fpirits.

F 4 Next

Next to thefe lingring durable pains, fhort intermittent, or fwift recurrent pains do precipitate patients into Confumptions; as lingring pains of the Stone, recurrent pains of the Stomach, Meagrims, and other forts of recurrent headaches do frequently mace-rate (*make lean*) the parts, and render their looks Confumptive and pining.

CHAP. XV.

Of an Aguifh Confumption.

AGues if deeply radicated (*rooted*) do frequently impell (*force*) bodies into Confumptions, by vitiating (*altering*) the Liver and Spleen, and perverting their Offices.

Among thefe, *Quartans* and *Tertians* of a long continuance do moft menace(*threaten*) this Symptom; the former as depending upon a corrupt incinerated (*burn'd*) melancholy, and the latter upon an adult (*burn'd*) *Stibial* or *Æruginous Sulphur* : both thefe being

being very active in devouring the fleshy parts, and intrenching upon the *fundamental mixture.*

A true and fimple *Tertian*, terminating according to the ordinary obfervation, in even returns or *Paroxyfms*, is now and then fucceeded by an *Hectick Feaver*, a fellow Symptom to a *true Confumption*, by reafon of its fwift termination, leaving fome deep relicks of its caufe (*viz. Stibial Sulphur*) in fome of the chief parts, where it lyeth clofely impacted (*propt in*) and is not eafily exter-mined (*removed.*)

Now, had the faid *Tertian* been of a more flow and gradual pace, it would gradually have expelled thofe Relicks; fo that you may know how dangerous it proves, for an Ague to difappear without taking Phyfick for it.

CHAP.

CHAP. XVI.

Of a Febril Consumption.

WE have oft observed, that malign
continual peracute (*very sharp and
violent*) Feavers do after moft dangerous
and doubtful attaques fuddenly remit into
fenfible abatement of the ardent (*burning*)
heat, infufferable thirfts, immanous (*raging*)
Head-aches and Phrenfies ; befides a change
of their low quick inequal Pulfes, into more
ordinate ones, and a mutation of their red
fiery Urin into a thick milky colour and
curdle fetling ; by all which appearances
hundreds of young Phyficians have been
deceived, and thereupon confidently affert-
ed their Patients free from all danger ; but
much to their fhame ; for thefe be certain
figns of an *Hettick* Feaver, and a true or
perfect Confumption, as appears by their
weak and languifhing condition, without any
fenfe of pain or heat, or perverfion of their
reafon

ſon, which may continnue ſo with them
r two or three weeks, and then they expire
e a waſted candle.

Moreover it's atteſted by many Phyſi-
ans, that a *Continent* Feaver, or a *Synochos
ſputris* doth ſometimes migrate (*change*)
to an *Hectick* Feaver.

CHAP. XVII.

Of a Verminous Confumption.

PHyſicians do ordinarily obſerve three
ſorts of Worms, engendred within the
ody of man, *viz.* ordinary Gut Worms
Lumbrici ſive vermes teretes)of a long and
lender ſhape like ordinary Earth Worms,
eing generated out of a ſlimy matter, col-
iquated from the Meſaraick Glandules and
dhering to the intern tumicks (*skins*) of the
hin Guts, which as ſoon as vivifyed (*grown
live*) through a vital ſpirit incloſed within
that ſlimy matter, as it were in a bag, and ſo
ſhaped into Worms, looſen and ſlide off
from

from the intern tunick (*coat*) of the Guts, and frequently creep into the *Stomach* for nutriment, being attracted thither by the sweet chyle (*the white juice of the Stomach,*) whence they are called Stomach or Mawworms. These being most usually engender'd in Children, do commonly cause them to look hollow-eyed with a lived (*of a lead Colour*) Circle about the under eye-lids, sharp nosed, thin jawed, and incommoded with a slimy mattery Cough, stink of Breath, and an Erratick Feaver; all Symptoms very near a kin to those of a *True Consumption,* and if not prevented in time render their Subjects incurable.

The cause of the foresaid extenuation of body and hollow-look, is imputed to the defect of nutriment, arriving through the chyle's (*the white juice of the Stomach*) being absorbed by the Worms, and the bloods vitiation (*alteration*) by malign putrid vapors, smoaking throughout the Vessels out of a putrefyed slime of the Guts, and so consequently rendred unapt of being apposed (*joyned*) to the parts.

The

The said putrid vapors through exciting a Feaver do colliquate the Phlegmatick humours of the body and brain, which transfuling (*sweating through*) or distilling to the Lungs, cause their mattery Cough.

The stink of breath is caused through steems, rising from the corrupted chyle of the Stomach.

There is a second sort of Worms, commonly resembled to a Womans hair-lace or fillet, thence called *Tænia* or *Tinea*, generated likewise in the Guts. The shape of these Worms is flat, small, and round, like to Gourd Seeds, which being link'd together to the breadth and length of an ordinary hair-lace, seem to be united into one intire Worm, which sometime is found to be of an incredible length, it may be of five or six yards, as *Tulpius* records in his observations. *Jacobus Oethæus lib. Observ. Med.* attests to have seen three Worms evacuated by a Woman, the longest whereof did equal Eighteen yards. *Alexander Camerarius* recites one of twenty yards long. *Platerus* reports a view of several Worms, that were at least forty foot long. The breadth

of

of this Verment is sometime an inch, othertimes half an inch broad. It appears usually
of an Ash colour, mark'd with black spots,
or cross lines going a thwart, dividing it into
thousands of small bodies like Gourds. Motion it hath none, so that it can scarce be
termed a moving creature, neither doth it
live, because it doth not increase internally
like living creatures, but by apposition.
So that it's called a Worm only from it's
external shape, and appearance, the head is
small and long, and the tail short.

Persons thus vermifyed (*troubled with
Worms*) seldome go to stool without avoiding a great quantity of those verminous
(*wormy*) seeds, and are oft incommoded
with gnawing griping pains round about the
Navil, oftimes extending to the Hip-bone;
which gnawing pains are apt to increase
upon the least emptiness of Stomach, so
that the patient is ever obliged to fill his Gut
with an immoderate proportion of food,
not only for to nourish his body, but also
to appease that ravenous Verment, which
notwithstanding doth defraude the body of
its nutriment, and infects the spirits with
malign

nalign steems, which in some space of time must necessarily produce a very sensible exenuation of the parts.

The material cause of this Worm is a vitious slimy chyle adured by a strong heat, that dryes it up into such numerous bodies.

Ascarides are a small sort of Worms ike Magots, bred in the *intestinum rectum*, or Gut of the Fundament, exciting an incommodious itching of the Fundament, with frequent desires of going to Stool. They are usually discovered by the excrements being perfused with them. This sort of vernent, immitting putrid fumes into the Vessels doth sometimes cause faints, and Convulsion Fits, as *Jessenus* witnesses to have seen such accidents in several. They may also by the same malign smoaks occasion a decay of the parts, though more rarely than Maw-worms or a *Tinea*.

These *Ascarides* do now and then creep into the Thighs and other parts.

Worms are likewise generated in most other parts of the body, though very infrequently. *Banhinus* (if I mistake not) speaks of a Worm generated in one of the Ventricles

tricles of the Heart, the patient dying of a Confumption. *Hollerius* reports a Worm difcovered in a mans Brain. *Duretus* remarks another generated in the Kidneys, and evacuated by Urin. Several make mention of Worms engendred in the Lungs, Liver, Spleen, *&c.* all perducing their fubjects into Confumptions.

CHAP. XVIII.

Of a Pockie Confumption.

THe ordinary back dore the Pox goeth out at, when it commits its fubject to the cuftody of its firft Mother Earth. is a Pockie Confumption, occafioned through the difperfion of virulent fteems out of the hearth of thofe Phagedenick Ulcers; by immanous *(outragious)* arthritick *(of the joynts)* pains, and continual vigilies *(intermiffion from fleep.)* But fince I have difcourfed of this in my *Venereal difcovery* fol. 167. and 168. I fhall infift no farther upon it.

CHAP.

CHAP. XIX.

Of a Bewitched Consumption.

Shall not here undertake the task of dif-
cuffing the poffibility of *fafcinous* (be-
tch'd) Difeafes farther, than refer your
nfures to fuch experimental inftances as
e produced for it. But whether thofe ex-
rimental remarques may be credited; and
fo, whether to be imputed to Witch-craft,
erein lyes the point of controverfie. Now
efe three Specifick notes will eafily refolve
e query.

1. The Symptoms of Witchcraft muft
infcend the dependance on natural caufes,
Vomiting Pins, pieces of Nails, *&c.*

2. There muft be feveral credible wit-
fs, that affert the fight of thofe fupernatural
mptoms.

3. The faid Symptoms, as they are fuper-
tural, fo they muft be only curable by
pernatural means, namely by Devout

G   Prayers,

Prayers, or Diabolical imprecations *(curſings)* and exorciſms, by the ſame or other Witches. Several there have been, that atteſted the ſight of perſons, that vomited Pins, Hair, Pieces of Nails, Feathers, *&c.* theſe certainly are ſupernatural Symptoms, if true; but thoſe witneſſes being ſuch, as their teſtimonies might well be doubted of, infer no concluſion.

2. it's certain ſome there have been that have vomited up the foreſaid bodies, but they were ſuch, as to get mony from the Spectators, had ſwallowed up thick ſhort blunt Pins, or Feathers, and vomited them up again voluntarily, as having a power to force themſelves a vomiting at their pleaſures by ſtraining, or by other means in taking Vomitories privately.

Theſe two Symptoms are generally aſſerted faſcinous. *(bewitcht) viz.*

1. A Lingring Conſumption without a ſenſible internal or external cauſe, and yielding to no kind of Phyſical Cure.

2. Effrayable and ſupervulgar Convulſio Fits, diſtorting the patients Neck and Bac in a manner, that it's a Thouſand wonder the

hey are not broken, or diflocated, turning
heir eyes e'en round within their heads,
eluding their Phanfies with ftrange fright-
il vifions, fpeaking ftrange languages, *&c.*
n emblem of the firft we have in the rela-
on of King *James* the 4. or 5. of *Scotland*,
tho falling away in his flefh more and more
very day, without the precedence of any
'rocatarctick caufe that fhould occafion it,
s Melancholy, ill Dyet, *&c.* and notwith-
tanding the helps of Phyfick againft any
ntern caufe or Difeafe, that might be ratio-
ially conjectured, at laft was fuddenly
ured by decharming the Witchcraft, that
hat had long been fufpected, and at length
lifcovered in *Danemark*, which was an
mage of Wax exactly refembling the faid
King, (whereby it was alfo known) and
iierced through in feveral parts of the body
vith pins, and particularly in thofe parts,
vhere the the King felt his pains, which as
hey were taken out of fuch parts, fo his
>ains ceafed likewife at the fame inftant in
he fame parts; and being all drawn out, felt
iimfelf intirely cured, and fuddenly grew
at again. In reference to the decifion of

this inſtance; there can be only this objected, that had the King taken no Phyſick, his Diſeaſe might more probably have been ſuſpected falcinous; but ſince he had made uſe of the beſt Medical helps the Art of man could afford, which continued for a long ſpace do oft at laſt perform marvailous cures; the Kings ſubitous recovery ought rather to be attributed to the Skill of his Phyſicians. Likewiſe Children are very apt to fall ſuddenly into a waſting of their fleſh, which happening as the other inſtance without any viſible cauſe, is frequently termed a Bewitch'd Diſeaſe; but queſtionleſs that Symptom muſt depend upon ſome obſtruction of the Entrails, or Verminous diſpoſition of body; and therefore a meer hallucination *(errour)* of the Vulgar.

The ſecond particular is exemplifyed in Hyſterick *(troubled with Fits of the Mother)* Women, eſpecially Maids, the rarity of whoſe Symptoms doth oft ſtrike ſuch an attonement into Spectators, that they confidently report them poſſeſſed with the Devil. In the year 1661. there lived one *Mary Waite* of the Society of Free-willing Baptiſts,

aptifts, at *Horly* in the County of *Oxon*,
ho was frequently troubled with miferable
ipes in her Guts, pinchings at her heart,
ioaking at her throat, fuppreffion of her
eath, blows on her head, ejaculations
om her feat, and fometimes off of the
orfes back whereon fhe rid, now and then
as ftruck dumb, deaf, and blind, oft enter-
ined with Angelick Vifions, and reduced
a very low ebb of Strength, *&c.* all which
:travagant Symptoms her Vifiters were
eafed to term Sufferings and Buffetings of
atan, and accordingly, to the intent of
rning this evil one out of poffeffion, they
ent near upon a Twelvemonth with her in
:ayer, but to little purpofe, until fuch
ne that one of her Vifions revealed to her,
at fhe fhould feed upon bread and water,
iild to a *Panada*, and drink nothing but
iring water; whereby fhe foon grew rid of
:r Devil, and intirely recovered. Now
iferve, to this day cannot that people be
:rfwaded, but that the forefaid *Mary* was
offeffed with the Devil, and afcribe her
:liverance to their implorations (*prayers;*)
that judging the nature of the Difeafe by

the

the remedy (*à juvantibus,*) if we believe
she was delivered from those Fits by Prayers of the Godly, we cannot deny the Disease
to be Diabolical *(of the Devil:)* But since
the case appears quite in another dress to
the eye of a Physician, who can soon produce
parallel Symptoms, if not worse, issuing
from ordinary Diseases, we may justly
doubt of the rise of this.

It's not rare to see young Amorous Girls
through the fury of an Hysterick *(Fit of the
Mother)* Paroxysme cast into a Trance for
an hour or two, and all that while under a
resemblance to the features of death; and
possibly diverted with some merry Phansies
or rare Visions of their Sweet-hearts, or of
Kings, Princes, *&c.* and it may be some a
Courting or Embracing of them, which makes
'em now and then burst out into a strange Fit
of laughing, to the amazement of their
Visiters.

Others again of a more zealous frame
during their Trance seem to converse with
nothing but Angels or Devils, as this foresaid *Mary,* who according to the Narrative
seems to have had several interviews and
dis-

scourses with Angels and Devils, the con-
nts whereof she afterwards recited to her
rethren, who faithfully recorded them
son Parchment, as some new Reve-
tions.

But those of a more trist *(sad)* and me-
ncholique composure, their Hysterick
rances proving Tragick perspectives to
em, perhaps of beholding the murder or
xecution of some of their dearest Relations,
those they bear an affection to, are inci-
nt into sudden cryes and howling tears.

And lastly, the Fits of others seems most
nergick in their tongues, in occasioning
em to speak strange Languages, and Sen-
nces like Oracles; to which latter some of
is age have given an equal credit, with
at of the Ancients to the Oracles of
elph.

It's inserted in Histories that a Maid of
iege, whilest detained with one of her
terin Passions, expressed her self very
nently in the *Greek* Tongue, although
hen released of her Fit, she was utterly
norant of the said Language.

G 4   Another

Another *Italian* Lafs *Peter Meffias*, &
Camerarius makes mention of in his *Hor.*
Succ. who proving Phrentick through the
extremity of a Feaver, fpake very goo
French, without ever having been known to
be experienced in that Tongue.　But to
return to *Mary*, wherein I do willingly re-
tard my felf fomewhat the longer, fince a
intire tract has been publifhed by her Bre-
thren to delude the world with their mira-
culous cafting out of a Devil ; which all the
while proved to be no other than an Hyfterick Paffion ; and if that may be termed a
Devil , then many an Hyfterick Woman
has a Devil more in her than fhe had before.

To render the point more clear ; her
choaking in her Throat , griping, and pinc-
ing of the heart, (*Cardiaca paffio*) her
trancing, imaginary beating of her head,
(which is no other than a fudden Convulfion
of the *Dura mater*) her being caft off her
Seat or Horfes back, an effect of a ftrong
Convulfion violently and fwiftly retracting
all the Mufcels of the body one way , which
muft needs be forcible enough to caft the
body to a great diftance ; for a man volun-

rily can caft his body a great way by leaping,
through the natural impulfe of fome of his
Mufcels , much more when they are all
violently moved one way by a ftrong Con-
vulfive motion; her ftrange vifions and
imaginations, *&c.* are all genuine Symptoms of an Hyfterick Paffion, or Fit of the
Mother , fuming up in malign and poifonous clowds to her Guts, and there caufing a
griping, thence to the mouth of the Stomach,
and there occafions that feeming pinching at
her heart ; thence to her Heart, where it
caufed a *Deliquium* (fainting) and *Syncope,*
(fowning) fo up to the Lungs , whence her
choaking ; and thence to the Brain, the occafion of all her depravate (*falfe*) vifions ; or
fometimes thofe venomous fumes might directly have tended to the brain, and fpring of
the feven pair of Nerves;& thence down the
back, where they may impell all the Nerves
and Mufcels into a Convulfion. Add hereto her cure by *Panada* , and drinking of
Spring water, (*argumentum à juvantibus*)
fingularly conducing to the repelling of thofe
uterin fumes, (*fmoaks of the Mother*) and
coarctating(*fhrinking*) the paffages, whereby
the

the said fumes muſt neceſſarily be intercepted, and in time abſolutely cure her.

However this one Symptom ſeems the
ſtrangeſt of all, that as ſhe rid on Horſeback
ſhe ſaw the Devil twice making to her in the
ſhape of a black Angel. As to this I am
very apt to believe her; and the manner
thus : her Imagination being depraved with
thoſe black Hyſterick ſmoaks, and accuſtom-
ed to receive an impreſſion of a Devil, from
thoſe black clouds forming themſelves into
ſuch a ſhape within the Cells of the Brain,
poſſibly juſt at the termination of the *Optick*
nerves , (*the Sinews of the ſight* ,) they
might eaſily return to the ſame ſhape and
impreſſion; beſides, thoſe clouds ſo ſhaped
might as wel make an impreſſion upon the
roots of the Optick Nerves within, which
continuated to the eye, eſpecially if hebetated
(*rendred dull or dozed,*) cauſe the ſame perception, as a wind within the head , when
the brain is diſtemper'd by a cold , beating
againſt the root of the auditory Nerve (the
ſinew of the hearing) and protracted to the
Tympanum (a little Skin within the Ear)
cauſes the ſenſation of a noiſe, as if it were
heard

heard from without, though it is not; or in short, why should not the Eye be subject to be deceived by an object from within, as well as the Ear by an internal noise, or the Tongue by a tast from within? that it is so, is apparent in Phrenticks, who do really imagine, they see that without, which their imagination is affected with within.

CHAP. XX.

Of a Consumption of the Back.

A *Consumption of the Back* here implyes little more than a sensible gradual diminution of the strength in the back, arriving through a counter-natural proflux (*flowing*) of *Sperm* (*Seed.*)

Common experience is a suffrage (*vote*) to *Galen's* Dictate, that a natural and moderate evacuation of Sperm through Venereal Embraces, doth greatly conduce to the preservation of health; disposes a man to fetch his breath more freely, and renders the body dy light and fprightful; and that not only in men, but other Animals; a Cock hath no fooner pleafed a Hen, but prefently after he Crows; a tone that correfponds to finging, attefting his mirth & fpritefulnefs:the reafon is becaufe *Omne nimium eft Naturæ inimicum*, whatever is overmuch is offenfive to nature, as opprefling the fpirits; which burden being diminifh'd, or taken off from them, muft needs render them more lively and lufty. Now the more noble and excellent that is, which is abounding, the greater damage it imports; and therefore blood when abounding, caufes acute putrid Feavers, inflammations of the Bowels, that oft inevitably tend to the ruine of the whole: but of a far more dangerous importance is an over plenitude of the Spirits, as being of a more noble and excellent degree; whence it is, that a retention of the Seed proves of fo calamitous a confequence, becaufe of its turgency with fpirits: in Women we fee it effects fuch effrayable Hyfterick Symptoms, (as appears in the Narrative of *Mary Waite*) as no other Difeafe can Parallel: in men it occafions inflammations of the Tefticles or Cods, (commonly

monly terminating into grangrenes, incurable
Ulcers,) a continual melancholick dull heavy posture of body, difficulty of respiration,
(*breathing*) palpitation (*beating*) of the
heart, a durable tinning noise and pains in
the head, and worse then all these a *Spermatick* (seedy) *Feaver*, in malignity and
putrefaction transcending all others. By the
way, this fort of Feaver is not mentioned by
any Authour, because it's comprehended
under continual humoral Feavers, but certainly for want of observation, whose Urins
if heedfully perspected, appear full of white
filaments (*threds*) or Spermatick Hairs,
which Physicians have hitherto erroneously
judged adust (*burn'd*) hairs expelled from
the Kidneys. Another most ridiculous(though
not without great danger) Symptom the said
Spermatick Plethory, or retention of Seed
produces in Women, is a Madness of the
Mother, (*furor uterinus,*) impelling them
to all manner of Lascivious looks, Bawdy
discourses, and inticing gestures, to such a
degree, that they oft take up their Coats,
and beg men to humour them, as if they
begged for an Alms.   Hereto corresponds

a

a *Madness of the Father*, which we find fo extravagant in fome men, that they cannot forbear, but mutt bend all their difcourfes looks, and actions, to wantonnefs; neither can this or that in Women be fentenced vice, becaufe occafioned by a Difeafe, which the Apoftle himfelf could term no other than *Burning*, (whereby we fee he compared it to the greateft pain in the world,) and therefore to prevent the growth of fo dangerous an accident, he advifed all rather to Marry than to Burn. However in thefe days that Symptom feldom arrives to that height of Madnefs in Men, fince they can eafily find the way to a Bawdy-houfe to prevent it; yet this doth not exclude but that its as poffible in them, as in Women, whofe chaftity worn into them by a ftrict education, rather than by the dictates of their feeble reafon, diverts them from taking the fame courfe of prevention. Neither is this all the mifchief of a *Spermatick Plethory*, oftimes tranfmitting hot putrid fteems of Sperm to the brain, (which is not ftrange, there being that Sympathy and intercourfe between the brain and the natural parts, that

the

he leaft Phancy of a pleafing object puts
hem into pofture,) which infinuating into
ts fubftance, engender a *Bedlam* madnefs.
And what makes fo many hundreds of Wo‑
nen run Mad, but that which they call *Love?*
y oft ftirring of thofe inflamed and putre‑
yed Spermatick fumes, which not being
ented through their natural paffages, are
reternaturally forced up into the pores of
he brain, whereby its temperament is fub‑
rerted, and a venene (*venomous*) quality
ubfequent to it, depraves the Phanfie into
a Madnefs. Now had thefe females not been
nterrupted with Wooers, thofe parts would
ave remained dormant, and confequently
iot attracted or generated fuch a quantity of
Sperm, which otherwife abounding and be‑
ng oft ftirred with their love vifions with‑
out evacuation, muft neceffarily putrefie.
So that we may hence plainly collect, the
firft inconvenience Women fall into through
rupture of Love, which had hitherto occa‑
fioned that plethory and commotion of
Sperm, muft be *Fits of the Mother*; becaufe
the Seed being augmented, moved, and not
vented, muft putrefie, and fo caufe thofe

Fit.

Fits.   2. The next inconvenience is a *Bedlam* madness (*mania*,) produced through a stronger passion of Love, occasioning a greater Plethory (*aboundance*) of Sperm and a stronger commotion, which not being vented, because of the Womans frustration in her Love, inflames and turns to a more malign venene putrefaction, whose fumes do easily intoxicate (*poison*) the Brain. Notwithstanding though all sorts of madness imply so difficult a cure, because of the deep latency of a venene cause in a noble part, yet this kind of madness that's occasioned by Love, in the commencement yeelds to the easiest cure, *viz.* by slackning the bridle of chastity, whereby vent is given to the putrefying Sperm, and the ascending malign Spermatick fumes revell'd (*drawn back:*) And by that sort of cure I have heard of several Women reduced to their perfect wits; and of two or three Maniacks (*Mad-men,*) who although impelled into that distemper through an adust malign *Hypochondriack* Melancholy, were set to rights again by the kindness of their Mistresses; for which cure there can no other reason be given, than that

Venereal

eneteal evacuations do potently revell (or
aw) from the head, (whereby the faid
elancholick fumes are retracted down-
ard,) and refrigerate *(cool)* the aduft hu-
ors that inflame the Brain; and laftly,
ate that over plenitude of raging fpirits.
loreover, we may obferve that *Italians,*
ough extremely difpofed to a Maniack
fadnefs, through their aduft Melancholick
:mperature and ftudious courfe of life, yet
's a very rare thing to hear of any Ma-
iacks among them, and that certainly for
o other reafon, than their frequent ufe of
Vomen, which the indulgence of their
.eligion has made Univerfal : on the con-
·ary in thofe Countreys, where the feve-
ity of their Laws doth ftrictly enjoyn cha-
ity upon the Inhabitants, as in *Holland,*
nough the coldnefs of the Climat and their
old Dyet doth oppofitely refift Maniack
Madnefs, yet there is not a Town fo fmall,
ut is provided with a *Bedlam,* for to fecure
hofe numbers of Maniacks both Men and
Women. Neither is the benefit of this fort
if evacuation fo particular, as to relate on-
y to individuals, but that the publick alfo

partakes

partakes of it, as in *Turky*, *Italy*, and *Spain*, and other Countreys, where *Polygamy* (having many Wives) and Scortation (*Whoring*) are tolerated, they find it renders their Subjects both Men and Women more tractable, and obedient to Government, and seldom are known to rebel; queltionlefs, by subtracting great quantities of spirits, which are fo copious in the Sperm, the Plethory whereof would otherwife render them (*viz*, the Spirits) turbulent and furious.

On the other fide where that kind of liberty is reftrained, their Subjects do oft fall into furies and rebellions againft the Magiftrate, as appears too often in thefe Septentrional (*northern*) climats: the reafon is as before, becaufe the faid Plethory, and retention of Sperm renders the Spirits furious and mad.

This premiffory difcourfe doth not infer fo great a dammage from an over-repletion of Sperm, but that the detriment of an over evacuation may be equal, or rather furmoun it. *Henricus ab Heer* in his obfervation relates the Cure of one of his Patients, who finding fuddenly reduced to the loweft eb of weaknefs, could fufpect no other caufe

bu

but his over-pleasing his Wife; in which
surmisal, the Patients Urin replenish'd with
whitish Spermatick Filaments, and his con-
fession after he had recovered his Speech,
confirm'd him. This doubtful Cure gave a
sufficient testimony of the danger, he was
precipitated into through that *Venereal
Syncope.*

Neither is this the sole Disease those furious Goats arrive to, but are oft strucken
with tremblings of the joynts, Palsies, Gouts,
and other neuritick (*Sinewy*) Diseases. Two
years ago, I had a *Flemmen* in Cure at *London*, his Disease was a Ptisick in a dangerous
degree, or *Asthma* oft excurring to an
Orthopnœa (*a Ptisick in the worst degree ;*)
the cause a *Metastasis* or translation of tartarous humours from his joynts to his Lungs;
for it seems his preceding Disease was the
Gout, which was droven inwards through
the unskilfulness of his Physician into his
breast. Hereupon I inquired into the first
occasion of this Arthritick (*of the joynts*)
malady, whether it was Hereditary, or
acquired by ill Dyet, or by what other external cause ; to this he gave me a full satis-

faction

faction, ingeniously confessing, that when a young man and marryed to a lusty *Frow* he had so travailed himself off his Legs, in yeelding to his Wifes insatiableness, that about a year after he fell into an Universal tremor *(trembling)* of all his joynts, that when going his Legs trembled under him, and was no sooner recovered of that, but Arthritick pains succeeded, which afterwards exchanged into an incurable Ptisick. Several other evils this kind of excess produces, but most frequently a *Consumption of the Back*, which *Hippocrates* stiles a *Tabes Dorsalis*, appropriating it most to youngmen, surfeiting themselves with the first tasts of their Nuptial *(wedding)* delights.

The immediate cause of this Consumption is an insupportable loss of Animal spirits *(those that move the joynts)*, engendred by the *Medulla Spinalis (or Marrow of the Back)* and the Brain, which said losse of spirits must necessarily occasion a great weakness of the Back and Brain, and consequently of all those parts that depend on them, *viz.* the joynts, as the Legs, Arms, &c.

2. The Brain and Back suffering so great a
draught

lraught of Animal fpirits, muft neceffarily
lraw a great proportion of Vital blood to
ecruit themfelves, and furnifh the other
)arts, that do fo immoderately draw from
hem, whereby the flefhy and other parts
)eing deprived of their nutriment, muft
:onfequently be extenuated, and if continu-
:d, reduced to a perfect Confumption.

That an exceffive evacuation of Sperm
loth fubtract fuch a large quantity of fpirits
$ plain to thofe, that conceive the genera-
:ion and conftitution of it; *viz.* it's con-
fituted and generated out of a copious
(plentiful) conflux *(flowing)* of Animal
fpirits, tranfmitted *(fent)* from the Brain
ind Marrow of the Back, through proper
:hanals, leading into the Tefticles, *(Cods)*
whofe office is to abftract the pureft part of
:hem, and fo to knit and unite them into
ı thick fluid body. Whence taking our Cal-
culation from the effence of wine abftracted
from its firft body, it appears probable,
that the Sperm being an effence abftracted
from a great quantity of Animal fpirits,
(which again are effences abftracted from a
large proportion of Vital blood) doth in the

H 3 quantity

quantity of a dram contain as many Animal
fpirits, as are contained in an ounce within
the Nerves, which ounce of fpirits can be
abftracted from no lefs than eight ounces of
Vital blood; if fo, you may eafily appre-
hend what dammage the body muft fuffer by
a fmall lofs of Sperm. That Sperm is ulti-
mately abftracted from Animal fpirits is
evident, in regard the Brain and Back do
fo immediately partake of the Symptoms of
an immoderate evacuation , *viz.* a great
weaknefs and pain of the Back, a contracting
pain of the Sinews in the Neck, and all the
Mufcles of the Body, and obtufion *(dulnefs)*
of the fenfes, both internal and external, *&c.*
I could infert many other arguments, clearly
demonftrating that affertion, but that my
compendious defign will fcarce permit.

To conclude , I fhall only add two ways
of immoderate evacuation of Sperm, *viz.* by
over-frequent converfes with Women ; and
by a Running of the Reins.

CHAP.

CHAP. XXI.

Of a Consumption of the Kidneys.

THe bare words of a *Consumption of the
Kidneys,* do plainly declare their pro-
er intendment, and therefore shall spare
ny pains of proposing a Description; that
which falls most in consideration, is the
aufes thereof, which may be conceived to
work that Symptom various ways, *viz.* by
starving of the Kidneys; by colliquation;
melting) by devoration or corrosion (*gnaw-
ng*) of their substance; or by dissolving of
heir fundamental mixture. In reference to
he first; they may be starved through obstruction of the *Emulgent* Vessels, that
hould transport their nutriment to them; or
hrough a compression and coarctation
(*shrinking*) of their substrance by reason of
ome compressing tumour within their flesh,
is a *Scirrus*, *Oedema*, or an Apostem, or
quantity of Gravel generated within their

Paren-

Parenchyma (substance,) or from a compressing cause from without, yet within their capacity or *Pelvis*, as a *Stone*, &c.

2. The humours and Fat of the Kidneys are apt to be colliquated (*melted*) through a great heat from within, as an Ardent (*burning*) colliquative (*melting*) Feaver, or an inflammation of their flesh; or through an excessive heat from without; as through over-riding, running, going, fitting with the back against a Fire, or against the hot Sun.

3. Mordicant excrementitions Gall, and Armoniack tartar ablegated (*sent*) thither with the Urine, do inflame, corrode, and Ulcerate their flesh, whereby it's converted into matter: or Gravel and Stone, generated within their capacity do oft grind away their flesh, and effuse their blood, apparent in a Sanguine Emiction (*making water.*) 4. Sometimes a malign humour insinuates into their substance, causing an immediate dissolution of their *Balsamick* principles, which happens now and then in malign Feavers; and by taking of poisons, as *Cantharides*, the Herb *Dipsacus*, &c. Through these kinds of Consumptions the

Kidneys

idneys have been obferved fome to be
ten away by an Ulcer to the ambient (*cir-
unding*) Skin, others to be dryed into a
iable (*brittle*) fubftance.

Each fort of thefe Confumptions is de-
ted by its proper Signs, *viz.* a colliqua-
ve Confumption by a great heat in the
per part of the Loins, a high coloured
rin with a number of fmall ftreeks of
t, fwimming a top in the form of a Cob-
eb. An Ulcer of the Kidneys is known
y a grating pain in the Loins, and
xcretion of matter, defcending to the
ottom of the Urinal. The other forts
re likewife diftinguifh'd by particular
gns.

CHAP.

CHAP. XXII.

Of a Confumption of the Lungs.

A Confumption of the Lungs may import two fignifications; the one, a confiderable wafting of the Lungs themfelves; the other, their occafioning the intire body to confume without any great lofs of their own fubftance. We fhall relate our difcourfe to both.

Reflecting upon the particular fubftance of the Lungs, their fituation, and connexion, (*faftning*) we fhall difcover them to be very much expofed to extern and intern injuries, and no lefs capable of injuring the Noble parts, whereby the whole by reafon of its abfolute dependance on them muft likewife receive a great prejudice. Anatomy exhibits the Lungs to be of a laxe, porous, light, or fpungy texture of fubftance, which wife Nature hath fo formed, for to anfwer her fcope, in a continual motion of infpiring and

expiring

piring the Air, whereunto a weighty body
ould otherwife prove very difobedient, and
nlefs porous and pervious (*full of holes*)
ke to a Spunge unfit to imbibe and tranfco-
te (*ftrain*) the Air ; for in effect the
fice of the Lungs is only to ferve the heart
n the capacity of Aereal ftrainers, to ftrain
he air and feperate it from grofs, or other
ffenfive inherents it may carry with it.
Vherefore fince the Lungs by reafon of their
ffice are obliged to a perpetual commerce
rith the Air, (which is fubject to momen-
ary alterations, now cold, hot, dry, or
noift, then thick, thin, foggy, rymy,
finking, poifonous,) they muft neceffarily
ye open to great yea irreparable dammages,
fpecially where their bodies are fo unapt
o refift or fuftain them, becaufe of their
hin, and lacerable (*eafily to be tared*) com-
pofure.

To thefe infpirable hurts we may annu-
nerate thofe they fuftain from their expiration of all fort of noxious (*offenfive*) and
fuliginous (*footy*) fteems, and ftinking putrid
breaths, and befides all that being conftantly
imployed in motion without acquiring

a

a moments reſt. Their ſituation is within
the breaſt, hung perpendicular under the
Brain, and near to the heart, whoſe wings
they repreſent, whereunto they are connect-
ed by the *Arteria Venoſa* and *Vena Arterioſa*; by means of which ſituation they are
expoſed to receive all the droppings from
the Brain, whence Coughs, Ptiſicks, Ulcers;
beſides the ill humours the *Vena Arterioſa*
conveighs thither, which together with thoſe
diſtillations from the Brain, finding them a
very fit Ciſtern, becauſe of their Sponginiſs,
do oft force them into ſuch a ſwelling, as
may juſtly be termed a Dropſie of the Lungs.
Next conſidering their coherence with the
heart, are thereby rendred more capable of
doing the greateſt miſchiefs.

By the precedence you may now obſerve,
how facil it is to drop into a Conſumption
of the Lungs, a Diſeaſe that is ſo fatal to
Londons Inhabitants; and no wonder, but
a greater wonder any can ſteal away into
their Graves without a Conſumption, conſidering the pernicious air of the City, the
weakneſſes of Lungs people inherit from
their Parents, and their expoſal to thoſe injuries, we have juſt now inſtanced.   CHAP

CHAP. XXIII.

Of the kinds of Pulmouique Conmumptions.

A Confumption of the Lungs is either without, or with an Ulceration. That without arrives through a Scirrofity, Apotem, Putrefaction of humours within its pores, or a *Crude tubercle* (*a fmall hard fwelling.*) 1. The Lungs oft imbibing Phlegmatique and Melancholique humours, (that are diftilled from the Brain, or conveighed thither through its pores and chanals,) are now and then deprehended Scirrous (*of a ftony hardnefs*) by diffipation (*difperfion*) of the fubtiler parts, and lapidification (*converfion into a ftony fubftance*) of the groffer that remain , or they may be left indurated (*hardned*) through the grofs reliques of a *Peripneumonia* , or inflammation of the Lungs. 2. By Diffection of expired Pulmonicks,(*difeafed in their Lungs*) their

their Lungs have oft appeared full of small hard Impofthums. 3. Excrementitious humours, such as are expectorated by a Cough after a Cold, or in an *Afthma* (*Ptifick*) *Peripneumonia*, or *Pleurifie*, are very apt to putrefie and corrupt in the Lungs, (as appears by the ftinking breath of fuch that are fo indifpofed,) whereby their acceffory nutriment being vitiated, (*rendred faulty*) and rejected by the Lungs, they are occafioned to waft. 4. A *Crude Tubercle* obftructing the infpiration of frefh air, and expiration of the fuliginous fteems of the heart, doth thereby extremely inflame and dry the Lungs, the continuation whereof doth at laft reduce them to an abfolute withering.

How thefe kinds of Confumptions propagate their evil to the whole body, ma eafily be collected from the former dif courfe.

CHA

CHAP. XXIV.

Of an *Ulcerous Pulmonique Consumption*

HEre I muſt make my Reader familiar with the Traditional notions, young ſtudents in Phyſick derive from their Hackney Authors, upon an Ulcerous Conſumption of the Lungs. And to be more methodical, it's not unneceſſary to digeſt their documents into ſeveral *claſſes*.

1. Let's make a diſquiſition of what they make of it. *Pulverinus, Godofred. Steeghius* fol. 447. and *Sennert.* 305. define it a Diſeaſe of a diminiſh'd bulk, (*diminuta magnitudo.*) *Hollerius, Duretus, Foreſt. Nic. Piſo,* &c. ſtate it a Diſeaſe of a diſcontinuated Unity, (*Soluta Unitas,*) becauſe it ſourceth from an Ulcer in the Lungs. *Platerus* paſſes it by, though *Mercurial* ſubtly ſpyes three ſorts of Diſeaſes in it, *viz.* a diminiſh'd quantity, a diſcontinuated unity, and a hot diſtemper.

diftemper. But *Capivac.* comments it chiefly
to be an hot diftemper, there being a continual heat of the parts, and an inflammation
of the Lungs, alwayes confpicuous in that
Difeafe. What to affert among thefe once
great *Rabbies* feems at firft fight difficult, but
upon a little panfing upon the matter you'l
find it a clear cafe. Thofe that infer a dif-
continuated Unity, namely the Ulcer in the
Lungs for the Difeafe, miftake the Difeafe
for its caufe, the Ulcer being the chief caufe
of the Confumption. Neither can they be
thought orthodox that fling in their verdits
for a *diminuted magnitude*, that rather appearing to be an effect, or fymptom of the
Ulcer in the Lungs, and fo is the heat of the
parts ; fo that none of 'em can hit one another in the teeth, that they are in the wrong.
But fhould I infift longer upon thefe triffles,
I am like to make my felf a participant of
their ridiculous difcourfes , and therefore
fhall ftep over to give you a brief of the
caufes, they allow to the forefaid Confumption ; though indeed I ought to have touch't,
what part they generally conclude the place
affected ; which fome will have the Lungs,
other

hers the heart, and many the whole body.
ie Authour of that Treatife intituled
e Definit. Medic. brings in likewife the
ealt, (*thorax*,) throat, and *afpera arteria*
ind-pipe) being affected with a malign
cer, for feats of an Ulcerous Confump.
m.

Touching the internal caufes of this fort
Confumption, Dogmatifts do univerfally
te an Ulcer of the Lungs to be the imme-
ate caufe, which happens fometime in the
arenchyma or flefh of the Lobes of the
ngs; othertimes in their pipes, (*bronchia*.
This Ulcer in the Lungs may be occa-
ned by feveral mediate caufes, *viz*.

1. Sharp bilious (*cholerick*) corrofive
gnawing) humours, iffuing out at the
res or lips of the veins, into the fpongy
bftance of the Lungs, whofe flefh they af-
rwards devour & corrupt, foon making a
utrid hole or cavern, which is then termed
n Ulcer of the Lungs.

2. *Hippocrates* affigns a *ferin* (wild and
ring) *Catarrh* falling into the Lungs, for
nother antecedent caufe of a *Pulmonique*
lcer: a *ferin Catarrh* is an hot, thin, and

I   fharp

sharp distillation of Rheum, which stream-
ing to the Lungs, gnaws their veins and flesh,
and so effects an Ulcer.

3. Gross Phlegm stagnating (*lying still*)
in the Lungs, in process of time putrefies,
and acquires a gnawing quality, thereby
making prey of the substance of the Lungs.

4. The rupture (*breaking*) of a vein in
the Lungs, effusing blood into their pores,
where it immediately putrefies and Ulcerates.

The Ulcer these causes produce in the
Lungs, *Hippocrates* calls a *ferin* (wild)
Ulcer, because the Nails of those, whose
Lungs are Ulcerated, are recurvated or
turn'd back like the claws of wild beasts,
that is, when they begin to draw near to
their long home.

Moreover this sort of Ulcer is ever cir-
rounded with an inflammation, which being
digested into matter, renders the Ulcer so
much the more sordid.

To these wee'l add two more, namely a
Pleurisie, which by expectorating (*spitting
out humors by coughing*) sharp putrid matter
through the Lungs, may now and then occasion an Ulcer.　　　　　　　　　　Lastly,

Laftly, an *Empyema* or a collection of
rulent matter in the capacity (hallow) of
e breaft, if not fuddenly cured, doth
doubtedly impel the Patient into a Phthi-
al Confumption.

Chymifts impute the caufe to a corrofive
lt, that's divorced from the *Sulphur* and
ercury of the blood, and afterwards dif-
lved in thofe liquors, that diftill into the
ungs.

CHAP. XXV.

*ontaining a difquifition upon the
caufes præcited.*

THe indexterity and worfe fuccefs of the
moft famous of our Confumption Cu-
rs, do evidently demonftrate their
imnefs in beholding its caufes; and upon
at account we may juftly prye into the
ayfteries they involve them in, and unravel
hat is fo ftrongly knit in every Phyficians
tricranium. To this purpofe we are to

gaze each limb of that Doctrine by it sel
under the aspect of these ensuing Queries.

1. *What kind of Choler this is that prov*
so ravenous upon the Lungs?

So careless are Authours in this particular,
that they imagine the cause of a Consumption sufficiently delared in their scripts, by
imputing it to excrementitious choler; but
whether they denote the ordinary yellow
gall, *(bilis flava) vitellin*, green, red, or
adust black choler, is left as a bone for every
Readers discretion to knabble at: if we should
commit the first of these, namely yellow,
or *vitellin* choler to the test, common observation in yellow Jaundises, and other Diseases excuses them from such an Ulcerous acrimony (*sharpness*,) wherein though very
copious and rampant, injure the body no
other way than by deforming it with a citri-
nous (*yellowish*) discoloration.

In the next place, yellow gall is so familiar with the substance of the Lungs, that
they seem to thirst chiefly after the more
yellowish or cholerick part of the blood for
their nutriture.

Green

Green gall the Institutists would persuade
, to be an effect of an over-hot Stomach,
oduced out of the hotter proportion of
e chyle, (*the white juice of the Stomach,*)
iich varies in deepness of colour, according
the intenseness of the heat of the Stomach,
me being of a lighter green like Verde-
ease, thence called Æruginous gall (*Bilis
Eruginosa,*) other of a deeper stain, or of
dark brownish green, like boyl'd Calwort
aves, or woad, thence termed *Bilis Glastea*;
iother of a green, different from both like
a leek, therefore denominated *Bilis Por-
icea*, i. e. Leeky gall. Neither is't their
idgment, that any of these greens should
e capacitated of damnifying the Lungs,
ecause of the remoteness of their harth; and
ras their Spring of a nearer situation, they
annot well tell how from a corrosive gall
o derive the other Symptoms, that usually
ttend Pulmonique Consumptives, as moist
Phlegmatique coughs, frequent spittings,
lrowsiness, and dulness of the senses; which
ather declare their dependance on a cold
Phlegmatick humour, than a sharp cholerick
me. Whence we may deduct a second and

third

third Query. *viz.* 2. *How chance fuch cold Symptoms in Confumptions to iffue from an hot caufe?* 3. Upon furmifal that Æruginous gall fhould gnaw Ulcers in the Lungs, *is it tranfmitted to them from the brain* (whether it may be fuppofed to be fublimed from the Stomach) *by diftillation, or through the Vena arteriofa? If either way, why fhould it pafs through the principal parts, as the Heart, or the Brain, without annoying either, which feem of a more tender difpofition than the Lungs, that are hardned with the weather, or extern air they infpire?* 4. It's wonder Authors never fummon'd *blew gall* for the caufe of Confumptions, which the expectorated (*fpit out by Cough*) matter oft appears tincted with; and beyond that, the Lungs of expired Confumptives do not feldome appear full of thofe blew kind of Spots, which inftance together with the eruption of blew fpots (*exanthemata livida*) in malign Feaver, are a certain atte of blew gall. This the Inftitutifts have f little noted, that they never thought o putting it in their Inftitutes. However no queftioning whether Green, Blew, or Blac

b

: the mifchief, fuppofing it to be any of
em, and fituated near or about the Sto-
ach, why fhould it prove more *Anarrho-*
us, (flowing upwards) fo as to attaque the
ungs, than *Catarrhapous,* (flowing down-
ards,)as it doth in a *Dyfentery*(bloody flux)
ins of the *Hæmorrhoids,* inflammation of
y of the lower parts, *Diabetes* (a conti-
ual piffing) or a hot *Dyfury* (difficulty of
aking water.) 5. *In what part of the body*
the true fpring, or fource, where this cor-
five choler is engendred? 6. *Whether a*
ulmonique Confumption never happeneth but
on fpitting or coughing up blood? 7. *By*
hat power or quality doth fleam ftagnating
the Lungs caufe a Confumption? 8. *Whether*
at confuming fleam is harbour'd in the
ipes, or fubftance of the Lungs within their
ores? 9. *Whether the foreinftanced fleam*
ftils from the head, or be imported through
e Veffels? 10. *Whether an Hettick Fea-*
r be a caufe of a Confumption, or a fymptom
the caufe of a Confumption, or fymptom of
e Confumption it felf? 11. *Whether a Pul-*
onique Confumption cannot happen without
e concomitance of an Hettick Feaver?

12. *Whether there be no other fort of true, perfect, or proper Confumptions, than a Pulmonique* (of the Lungs) *Confumption?* Thefe and many other problems being paffed by, not only for ftating of them, but refolving, do impeach Phyficians of their floth, and abfolute infufficiency of curing Confumptions, which unlefs determined is a pregnant teftimony, they manage their office in that Difeafe with as little Skill as Confcience. Neither is the reader to behave himfelf fo ftrict and precife as to be contented with no lefs clear a folution than a demonftration, our notions in Phyfick being of that fcantnefs, as feldom reach beyond a rational conjecture; which if I ingaged to remonftrate here in this Chapter, fhould in order of difcourfe be obliged to make ufe of the terms and principles inferted in this and the preceeding Chapter, and that with the fame difadvantage other affertions have hitherto fo obfcurely been proved. Wherefore I fhall refer you to the next enfuing Chapter, where I do expect a grain's or two allowance, which all men have granted them

in

attempting a folution of doubts by them-
lves ftated.

CHAP. XXVI.

*f a more apparent caufe of a Pulmo-
nique Confumption.*

THE paffage to this abftufe (*hidden*)
fpeculation is like a Labyrinth (*maze*)
livided into feveral ftops, turnings or wind-
ngs, where at each divifion we muft halt,
o advife what way lyes moft direct whither
ve are defign'd; for the truth of caufes fteps
o lightly through mens imaginations, that
they muft ufe great fubtility to track its
veftiges (*footfteps,*) which we find now
adayes fo obliterated (*blotted out*) with
their courfe fearches, that it feems almoft
barricado'd from any intellectual approach.
In purfuit of this precept wee'l advert you
of feveral ftops or windings, being neceffary pofitions, whofe light will lead you to
that fo obfcure caufe of a Confumption of the
Lungs.   *Thefi-*

Thesis 1.

Symptoms impreſſed by corroſion point at corroſive bodies for their cauſes. In Pulmonique Conſumptions the preternatural concomitants (*attendants*) *viz.* an univerſal heat of the body, an Hectick Feaver, a torminous diarrhé, (*griping looſeneſs*) acre (*ſharp*) and hot diſtillations, &c. have all a ſtamp of a *Corroſive* (gnawing) quality, and conſequently are introduced by a corroſive humour.

Thesis 2.

There are but two ſorts of corroſive humours engendred within the body of man, namely, *Choler* and *Melancholy*; And between theſe the impute of a Conſumptive cauſe will lye. Touching Fleam, and that they ſingle for pure blood, neither can be imagined participant of acrimony, but rather demulcers, and qualifyers of it. Which of the two abovementioned corroſives is the chief actor here, the following poſitions will reſolve you.

Thefis 3.

Choler is the lighteft, and moft inflamma-
part of the blood. Whence namely from
inflammability its refembled to, and call-
a *Sulphur.* This pofition informs us of a
lgar errour, terming the gall bitter, as
eir proverb more peremptorily implyes,
's *as bitter as Gall;* whereas in effect,
ere's nothing guftable, fweeter; for what
moft inflammable muft be moft unctuous,
t and oyly, nothing being apter to take
ame than Oyl, Fat, Butter, and other
ctuous bodies; and what is moft oyly and
ctuous muft needs partake of a fweet fa-
our, namely, of a fat fweetnefs, which
hyficians term *Pingue dulce,* or a fat fweet;
d of that guft is the Gall or Choler, being
e flower and butter of the Blood. This
ppears more evident in milk, which is
othing but blood turned white, by being
iluted *(water'd)* with a greater quantity
f *Serum* or whey, (that is a certain wate-
ifh liquor floating in the Veffels) in the
Glandules *(Kernels)* of the breaft; now milk
eing charned in a Tub vomits up it's butter,
which

which is that light and inflammable part reduced to its native colour, and above termed Gall.

Thesis 4.

Choler is in it self refistent of having any kind of bitternefs extracted, or produced out of it ; no, not by any kind of inflammation. If any force will imprefs fuch a bitternefs, as is thought to be in choler, it muft be by aduftion *(burning)* or putting it into a flame, which is fo far from admitting an Empyreume *(burning,)* or conceiving any bitter afhes, that confifting of a pure oyly nature, when fet in flame , it burns clear away without leaving any cindars or aduft matter, to atteft its latent *(hidden)* bitternefs; as doth more plainly appear in Butter, Tallow, or Oyl, burning away in a Lamp, without leaving any thing bitter behind them.

Thesis 5.

What amaritude *(bitternefs) or acrimony* (fharpnefs) *is deprehended in Choler, it acquires from a commixture of Melancholy, or extern malign bodies imported with the air.*

Th

...s Thefis is a neceffary confequence of the
ext preceding; for if gall cannot be rendred
crimonious *(fharp)* or bitter of it felf, nor
y inflammation; than neceffarily whatever
crimony or amaritude at any time redounds
n it, muft be derived from the admixture
of another fharp bitter fubftance, which
among the humours can be no other than
Melancholy; Phlegm and pure blood, be-
ng reputed allayers of acrimony, and upon
that account *Avicen* countermands letting
blood in cholerick bodies, becaufe he efteems
the blood (which he chiefly here intends
pure blood and Phlegm) a *franum bilis,*
or a bridle of the Gall, obtunding *(dulling)*
its acrimony and fiercenefs.

Thefis 6.

*Choler being fet in fire, and acting upon
Melancholy, or rather calcining it into fmall
acuated (* fharp pointed) *minimal bodies, is
by their incorporation with it felf, rendred
acrimonious and bitter;* whence I conclude
Choler accidentaly bitter and acrimonious,
but not in it felf.

This bitternefs and acrimony varies in
in-

intenseness and remisness, according to the degree of calcination of Melancholy, and proportion of Choler it is admixt to.

Thesis 7.

Choler by the premisses is evidenced of being capable only of flaming and kindling a Feaver in the body ; and consequently Melancholy calcined by the flames of Choler must remain the sole cause of acrimony, and corrosion, and inclusively of occasioning Ulcers both within and without the body.

Thesis 8.

The heart beating vigorously and strong, doth together with its *Sulphurous flames* expell the foresaid calcined melancholy to the circumference, especially if the said humour be but diluted (water'd) with the serosity (waterish liquor) of the blood. Neither is this sole vital faculty sufficient to exterminate (*turn out*) noxious humours to the periphery or outward parts, unless the animal faculty be concurrent with it, to supply the Fibres with Animal Spirits, which do not only render them strong to expel, but sensible

of

f feeling the leaft fting of any offenfive
imour, whence they are immediately
rick'd or fpurred to contract themfelves,
id by means of that contraction to expell.
on the contrary the heart beats weak, and
ie animal faculty be found faintifh, the
orefaid acrimonious humour remains within
nd caufes internal erofions.

Moreover, notwithftanding the ftrength
f both faculties, the humours expelled to
he circumference, are apt now and then to
egurgitate (*flow back*,) by reafon of ob-
tructions in the capillar (*very fmall like
iairs*) veins, terminating in the extreme-
ies.

Hitherto we have difcourfed of the fame
aufes, how they happen to engender feve-
al Difeafes, though in the fame bodies, but
it different times.

That which falls next in confideration, is
in anfwer to the fourth Query of the Chapter
oreceding, viz. *Why the fame corrofive humour fhould fometimes prove* Anarrhopous
(*flowing upwards,*) *and generate Difeafes in
the upper parts; and otherwhiles* Catarrhopous
(*flowing downwards,*) *impreffing maladies
npon the lower.* The

The occasion of the various diversion of the foresaid humour is situate partly in the disposition of the part *Mandant*; the strength and weakness of the vital and animal faculty; the parts *transmitting*, or giving passage; the disposition of the part *recipient* (*receiving*;) and the qualification of the humour *transmitted*.

The part Mandant (*sending or expelling*) is here chiefly intended for the place, where this acrimonous humour is generated, and harth or spring, whence it sourceth and erupts.

The place is, where the acrimonious (*nourishing*) humours are primarly (*first*) concocted, or receive the form of humours, and where they are afterwards further wrought, purifyed and clarifyed. This assertion probably will accuse many parts more, than what ordinarily Physicians have their eye upon.

The Stomach is a part that primarl digests, and converts Victuals transmitte thither, into a whitish or cineritious (*li ashes*) humour, called the *Chyle*, which i it be not exactly dissolved into an eve thoroug

orough melted juice, muſt neceſſarily
ound with thick and groſs admixtures.
ow, it's a current ſaying among us, that
e fault of the firſt concoction or digeſture
not amended in the ſecond, (*vitium pri-
æ coctionis non corrigitur in ſecunda;*)
herefore the chyle being tranſmitted crude
d groſs into the Veſſels, and arriving in
e Spleen and Liver, ſticks in the capillar
ins, and keeps in the heat or hot ſteems
at ſhould ariſe out of their *Parenchyma*
r fleſhy ſubſtance) to ferment attenuate,
d defæcate (*clarify*) the blood. The heat
f thoſe entrails being thus incloſed and pend
p, redoubles, and gradually after it hath
tremely dryed and ſcorched, burns and
alcines them into a kind of fixt Salt, which
cording to the nature of the Victuals,
vhence they received their conſtitution)
d the intenſion of heat, proves a *Nitrous,*
Vitriolat, or *Armoniack* Salt. The Spleen
a this caſe is found to contain a Mine more
equently producing an *Armoniack*, and
Vitriolat Salt, with a ſmall admixture of
coagulated *Sulphur.*

The Liver is the more fertil parturient of

K   Nitrous,

Nitrous, and sometimes of a *Vitriolat* and
Armoniack tartar, but with so copious a
commixture of coagulated (*thickned*) choler
or *Sulphur*, that it ought rather to be named
a *Cinnabrin or Æruginous Sulphur*, from the
greater proportion of *Sulphur* to a far smaller
of Salt. The heart we conceive to be the
sole mine of *Arsenical Sulphur*, whose pernicious steems insulting upon the Vital Spirits, produce malign and spotted Feavers.

The Stomach is likewise oft stuff'd between its tunicks (*coats,*) and in the smaller
branches of Vessels, that are inserted into
its body, with the dregs of obstructive crude
chyle, whereout such Salts and Sulphurs are
calcined and extracted, as in acrimony and
corrosion prove no wise inferiour to those
engendred in the Spleen or Liver, since
produced with so intense a heat as is required
for the first solution of the hardest food; and
probably a stronger heat, being raised to a
higher pitch by obstructions, and the ebulli-
tion of some of those acrimonious bodies
already engendred.

That the Stomach is so common a spring
of Consumptive sublimations and distillations,

ons, needs no other proof, than the fenfe
the Patient, attefting a great clog and
preſſion at his Stomach, oft crying out, if
at were removed, he ſhould be well;
ſides his nauſeouſneſs, vomiting, and diffi-
lty of digeſture, he finds his gulſet all along
ry ſore, rough, and ſtuffed with humours,
bliming upwards, which ſometimes may
t reach ſo high as his brain, but are imbi-
d by the tonſils and other Glanduls about
e Throat, where in like manner aforeſaid,
ey are diſſolved into an oyl, and ſo diſtill
tween the Membranes of the *Aſpera*
teria into the Lungs. To this the reme-
es (*argumentum à juvantibus*) add an un-
ieſtionable verdit; Vomitives being twice
: thrice exhibited in the beginning or aug-
ient, do oft eradicate the mineral cauſe of a
onſumption. Likewiſe *Lohocks*, and Syrups
nt are ſo uſually preſcribed, do immediately
em to abate and demulce the hoarſeneſs
d violence of a Cough, by mollifying the
iggedneſs of the intern tunick of the Gullet,
nd thickning or rendring the matter of the
ough, that aſcends upwards between the
unicks of the foreſaid *Oeſophogus*, more glib

K 2 or

or flippery. So that we muft not imagine,
that Syrups or other expectoratives do ad-
advantage in Coughs, by flipping down between the *Epiglottis*; for as I inftanced before, that muft neceffarily occafion a greater
Cough, and difficulty of refpiration. Neither is't probable they circulate about to the
heart and *Vena arteriofa*, to arrive to the
Lungs; for before that time their fweetnefs
whereby they are fuppofed to lenifye a
Cough, and other vertues, would be obtufed
and altered into other qualities; or if we
fhould admit that fuppofal, they could not
be thought to auxiliate the Cough in fo fhort
a fpace as they do.

Having now given you a divertifement
in declaring the parts *Mandant*, we are to
proceed in illuftrating, whence the faid
falin and fulphurous productions receive
their direction or firft motion, that renders
them *Anarrhopous*, not paffing by to indigi-
tate (*point*) at the parts *Tranfmittent*.
Wee'l fuppofe the Spleen the chiefer of the
two harths, or parts *Mandant*, and principally obftructed in its lower parts and Splenick branch, whence a potent heat breaking
forth

rth caufes the *Orgafmus* (a fwelling fer-
entation) to boyle or tend upwards, or
ther fublimes the forementioned calcined
lts through the Arteries up into the right
entricle of the Heart, where having
ffed another reverberation are propelled
to the Lungs through the *Vena arteriofa.*

Moreover we muft likewife allow a fmall
mmixture of *Sulphur* to the Salts, which
th not only contribute a force to the calci-
tion, but a facility to the fublimation.
his fixt *Vitriolat* or fometimes *Armoniack*
lt being impelled into the pores of the
pungy flefh of the Lungs, meets there with
ferofity, or waterifh kind of moifture,
iffolving it immediately into an *Oleum per*
eliquium, (an oyly liquor) like other cal-
ined Salts are apt to do, when they arrive
any waterifh moifture, as being put
a Cellar, or placed over warm water.
he falt now turned into a corrofive liquor
r oyl, is rendred capable of penetrating
piercing) into the fmalleft and deepeft
ores of the Lungs, whofe flefh it foon dila-
erates (*tares*) and gnaws into an Ulcer;
nd not only fo, but being indued with a

K 3   quality,

quality, all other calcined Salts are (as you may experience by holding Allom or Salt-peter in your mouth) of attracting and raising fleam and moisture out of the Lungs and other parts adjacent, doth continually incite the Lungs, to avoid great quantities of spittle, fleam, and other sharp stinking matter by Cough.

Lastly, the Stomach as it first sowed the Seeds of this evil, so it continues likewise to foment them, and act the part of another chief *Mandant*; and in some it's found to be sole and principal; which as I expressed before, being stuffed in its tunicks, obstructed in the inserted Vessels, and clogged round about with a weight of acrimonious humours, doth likewise glow with a strong heat, whereby the said salin accumulation (gatherings or heaps) are sublimed, according to the length and direction of the intern and extern membranes of the *Oesophagu* (*or gullet*) to the brain, by whose waterish moisture it's likewise dissolved into an *oleum per Deliquium*, (*or liquor like oyl*,) which through its attracting and raising of liquo doth overwhelm the brain with fleam an moistur moisture, whence becaufe of its weight and pricking, it's continually præcipitated into the Lungs, *viz.* according to the direction and longitude of the membranes, down into the *afpera arteria* (wind-pipe,) that is be-tween its membranes, not through the *:pyglottis (the grifly cover of the wind-pipe,)* for that would immediately fet the patient a Coughing. Thus a ferin Catarrh happens, which through its corrofive(*gnawing*)quali-ty oft Ulcerates the Lungs; efpecially if fe-conded by thofe Salin fublimations from the Spleen.

Neither is the Liver alwayes excufable, now and then tranfmitting a *cinabrin Sul-phur*, through the *Vena cava* to the Brain, or Heart, and thence to the Lungs, being likewife generated by a reduplicated heat, occafioned through the obftructions of its Capillars (fmall veins like hairs,) and branches that tend to the Gall Bladder. So that hereby the Spleen more frequently and principally, next the Stomach, then the Liver, do demonftratively appear to the parts *Mandant*; the Brain, Heart, *Thymus*, Glandules of the Gullet, and Tonfils the

parts

parts tranfmitting, or only giving paffage to the humours forced up thither from other parts.

Here you may take notice of a grand errour among Practitioners, opinionating the Brain the chief part *Mandant*, when diftempered with a cold humorous intemperament, and diftilling into the Lungs: and of this finifter fentiment are they fo confidently poffeffed, that they bend all their prefcripts and devifes to dry up this fountain of Rheum, to which purpofe *Crato's* Amber Pils, *Fonfeca's* Decoction of Sanders, *Eraftus* his Dyet Drink of *Guaiacum* and *Salfa*, abforbing Emplafters to be applyed to the head, Fontanels (*Iffues*,) Ventofes (*Cupping-glaffes*,) Veficatories (*Emplafters to draw Blifters*,) and Phlebotomy (*opening a Vein*) are all fummoned in as *Herculean* auxiliaries (*helps*,) to dry the Brain, but rather the purfe.

Another opinion they are very fond of, is, that the internal part of the *Afpera arteria* (wind-pipe) is the part tranfmittent, an abfurdity every drop that goes down the wrong way will confute. What other ridiculous

ulous tenents they foment touching Ca-
arrhs, were a fhame to recite to fuch as
now better things.

How the Vital and Animal faculties
prove accidental occafions of this evil,
hrough their faintnefs, whereby they are
ncapacitated of propelling thofe noxious
(*offenfive*) fublimates downwards, is apo-
liftically expreffed in the beginning of the
eight *Thefis*, (pofition) and therefore wee'l
fuperfede the needlefs pains of a repetition,
only wee'l add the pofitive concurrence of
the Animal and Vital Spirits in directing
and derivating (*drawing*) the forefaid fublimates to the heart and brain; namely,
encountring with each annoying and pernicious effumations (*fmoaks*,) are compelled
to a retreat to their Spring head, whither
they do likewife conduct thofe Salin fteems
along with them. The *Recipient* part is the
Lungs, who are partly paffive in being forced to receive, and partly active in attracting fuch corrofive Salts. Their fituation and
connexion obliges them to receive the precipitates from the Brain, Heart, and Stomach; their acts of expiration (*breathing*
out)

out) attract potently from the Veins, Arteries, and other parts, as appears in those fuliginous *(footy)* smoaks, and putrid steems they expire. What doth further dispose them to a neceſſity of receiving thoſe ſalts, and other malign humours, a repeated Survey of Chap. 22. will aboundantly ſatisfie you.

The qualification requiſite in the humour tranſmitted *(viz.* the deſtilled liquor*)* may eaſily be deduced from the premiſſes; namely, a degree of acrimony wrought into a tartarous humour by calcination, reaching at leaſt to the aſcent of a Vitriolat, if not an Armoniack Salt.

By the way take this for none of the leaſt important remarques, that this liquor, that's produced out of the ſolution of a Vitriolat Salt ſublimed to the Brain, if accidently it ſhould penetrate into the concave of the Nerves, (as it would eaſily do, ſince conſiſting of a ſharp ſalin thin inſinuating ſubſtance, were it not diverted by being precipitated into diſtillations,) it ordinarily cauſes Convulſions and Epilepſies *(the Falling Sickneſs.)*

                                    The

The Second, Third, and Fifth Problems
being all refolved in the contents of the folution of this fourth, wee'l ftep over to the
fixth ; *Whether a Pulmonique Confumption
never happeneth but upon fpitting or coughing
up blood ?* Galen and his Cotemporaries did
commonly obferve Pulmonique Confumptions to follow a fpitting of blood, whence
many of his Sectators do ftill perfift in the
fame tenent, not confidering, that what was
ufual in *Galen's* time may be lefs common
now ; for Pulmonique Confumptions do as
frequently appear among us here, that are
molefted only with an acrimonious moift
kind of Cough, as thofe, that have fallen
into that evil upon fpitting of blood, hapning upon a rupture, or corrofion of a vein
in the Lungs.

Befides my own fentiment, I'le infert the
obfervations of *Argenterius* and *Fernelius* ;
The former in his *Comment.* 3. in *Art.
Medic.Gal.* gives a relation of four women,
that dyed all of exquifite Ulcerous Pulmonique Confumptions, none whereof coughed up blood.   And *Fernelius* writes thus :
Some upon the fpitting only of a liquid and
yellowifh

yellowish humour, being taken with a small Feaver, have begun to consume, and a long time after did spit a little blood mix'd with matter; but I have likewise observed a many that dyed Consumptive, in whom there was not not the least appearance of blood through-out their whole sickness.

Moreover, observe there is an Ulcerous disposition of the Lungs, and an Ulcer of the Lungs; And both these may be appositely termed causes of a Pulmonique Consumption, or Consumption of the Lungs. By an Ulcerous disposition of the Lungs, I intend a perfusion of acrimonious salin liquors (such as I instanced before) throughout the body of the Lungs, insensibly drying, gnaw-ing, and absorbing their flesh, and likewise insensibly dissipating it into vapours and ex-halations through the pores of the *Parenchy-ma*, and ambient Membrane; which latter though *Galen* denyes to be pervious with a number of small holes, is found to be so by *Aristotle*'s and others experience.

Thus the Lungs of many deceased Con-sumptives have been discovered quite con-sumed, nothing remaining but the ambient
(cir-

cirrounding) Membrane (*skin*,) and a umber of withered veins and filaments *thred*;)without the precedence of fpitting f blood or matter.

Moreover as I obferved in Chap. 23. Confumption of the Lungs may alfo arrive pon a fcirrofity, hard Apoftems, (as *Atheoms, Steotoms,* &c.) putrefaction of humours within its pores, and a crude tubercle, or drying fcorching fuliginous fteems continually fuming from the heart , without the leaft appearance of expectorated blood. In this particular I remember one of our elderly *Oxford* Phyficians proved difappointed of his Prognofticks, or rather Diagnofticks. A Scholar applying himfelf to him for information, whether he were in a Confumption, was anfwered with a queftion, whether he fpitted blood ? whereat the Scholar replyed negatively; than faid he, 'tis but a Ptifick Cough, and I'le warrant you from a Confumption, though three months after he left a *Skeleton* behind him, to witnefs what he dyed of.

The Seventh, Eighth, and Ninth Query you'l find folved by what is declared already.

The

The Tenth is, *whether an Hectick Feaver be a cause of a Consumption, or a symptom of the cause (*Symptoma causæ*) of a Consumption, or a Sympom of the Consumption it self, (*symptoma symptomatis ?)* Certainly it's a symptom of the cause, and a fellow symptom with the Consumption of the intire body.

The Eleventh demand is, *Whether a Pulmonique Consumption may not happen without the concomitance of an Hectick Feaver?* This I may safely conclude, there is many a Pulmonique Consumption without the evident signs of an Hectick Feaver, *viz.* a sharp equall heat over the whole body, a glowing of the extremities an hour or two after meat, a quick low pulse, &c. without which I can attest, I have found several Consumptives, though for what I knew, there might very probably have been a latent (*hidden*) Hectick. Howver for the most part there is a sensible *Hectick* attending Consumptives. But out of this discourse there may be a very important question started, Whether that Hectick Feaver be a *Morbus in esse* (a Disease already generated,) r a *Morbus in fieri* (a Difeafe in engenring? If we fuppofe it a *Morbus in effe*, ian though the Ulcer were dryed up and ared, the Hectick would remain, as being Fire kindled out of the *Innate heat* and *Radical moifture* into an actual flame, and epending upon no fewel but its felf, which rould continue burning until the *radical* moifture were burn'd away. On the other and, if we confider it as a *Morbus in fieri*, han it muft have its dependance upon purulent fteems difperfed from the heart togeher with the blood to the parts, where rriving they caufe a kind of heat and glowng in the fubftantial principles, whereby hey are fet in fire, until the purulent acrinonious fteems are diffipated. The fympoms make this appear very probable, *viz.* a glowing heat being a new fermentation two iours after victuals, excited through the ippelling purulent corrofive fteems, tranforted thither with the blood. 2. The Pulfes confirm the fame inference, changing quick, hot, and acre *(biting to the touch)* at the advent *(coming)* of the forefaid fteems; and after a while when they are confumed

and

and expelled by tranfpiration, they return to a more moderate motion, until the next flood of fermenting matter.   3. Were this affertion not admitted, that the forefaid Pulmonick Hectick is a *Morbus in fieri,* than neceffarily an Hectick once kindled would impell the patient into a Marcour, though the Ulcer in the Lungs were cicatrized; the contrary whereof hath been difcovered in feveral; fo that you may reft certain, that the Ulcer being cured, the *Hectick* vanifhes with it.   Hence you may extract, what I intend by an *Hectick Feaver,* namely the *Innate heat* kindled into a deftructive fire, violently abforbing the oyly *Radical* moifture, through the appulfe of falin fteems, which through their contrariety to the Balfamick mixture excite a fervent fermentation in this latter, like oyl of Vitriol, powred upon oyl of tartar, or water upon lime.

Laftly, wee'l conclude Ulcers that fucceed the burfting of a Vein in the Lungs, and fome others induced by other caufes, to depend for a confiderable time, before the can attain to that height of exciting a Hectick Feaver; for we cannot fuppofe th

Hea

ſeart to conſiſt of ſo ſmall a force, as not
ɔ be able to reſiſt thoſe purulent fumes
or a while, and divert them from the other
arts, into whoſe Penetrails *(depth)* to in-
inuate, ſome proportion of time muſt be
llowed.

.. The Twelfth and laſt Interrogatory is ,
Vhether there be any other ſort of true, per-
ect, exquiſite, or *proper* (for thoſe terms
ıre reciprocately uſed by Authors) *Conſump-*
ions , beſides a Pulmonique Conſumption ?
This Query implyes rather a controverſie
ıbout words , than the thing it ſelf ; for
if they reſolve to term no other an exquiſite
or proper Conſumption, but a Conſumption
of the Lungs,(words being to be underſtood,
ex intentione imponentis, from the intention
of him that impoſes the word,) then the
caſe needs no debate ; but if the words are
ɩo be taken (*ex apprehenſione intelligentis*)
from the apprehenſion of thoſe that under-
ſtand, or whom they are ſpoken to , then
the regiſter of Conſumptions will be much
enlarged. Now ſo it is, that the common
intendment ſtates a proper Conſumption ,
a diſſolution or corruption of the Balſamick

principles ; and confequently if differencing perfect Confumptions by the variety of their caufes, and feats of thofe faid caufes, we muft infer many more, as an *Hypochondriack*, *Amorous*, *Ulcerous*, *Cancerous*, *Renal*, *Dorfal*, and many other forts of Confumptions before commented upon.

If probably I have not propofed refolves to thefe Queries, that are enough feafoned for every Readers palat, I muft beg his excufe upon pretence, it's but the firft rough draft, which upon a fecond attempt may be rendred better polifh't : However fuch as they be, they'l prove a more luminous and foveraign Directory for the Confervative, Prefervative, and Curative part of a Confumption, than any hitherto offer'd to view.

CHA

CHAP. XXVII.

fome lefs frequent and rarer caufes
of a Pulmonique and other forts of
Confumptions.

"O decline confufion of caufes we have
referved thefe ; being of a more rare
ergency, for a particular remarque. This
tinction of Confumptions is univerfally
erved, that fome are moift, others dry.
moift Confumption receives its nomen-
ture (*name*) from a moift fputation
pitting) or expectoration that attends it;
ry one is known by its dry Cough : This
ter, befides the ordinary præcited caufes,
fometimes occafioned by various acci-
ts of the Heart, as Wounds, Ulcers,
nes, Stones, and Worms, that are bred
it, and particularly by a *Marcour*, or a
ttick of the Heart, which together with
Lungs, as *Melangthon* witneffes (*lib.* 1.
Anima) were found to be as dry as a

L 2   Baked

Baked Pear, in the expired body of *Cafimir*
Marquéfs of *Brandenburgh*.   Thus likewife
Telefius reports the heart (and confequently
the Lungs) of a noble *Roman* dryed away
by an immoderate heat, to nothing but the
skin. *Fernelius* in his *Pathol. lib.* 5. *cap.* 12
tells us of one that dyed Confumptive,
whofe heart was afterwards difcovered to
be corroded into three large Ulcers, the
fteems of whofe matter muft needs have
infected the Lungs. *Bauhinus* among hi
obfervations regifters this following; that
he diffected a Corps, wherein he found the
Lungs confumed; the capacity of the breaft
to be full of putrid and concreafed blood,
the *Pericardium* (a skin wherein the heart
lyes inclofed as in a bag) to contain above a
quart of white matter (*pus*,) and the heart
extremely extenuated and confumed about
the furface. The fymptoms that molefted
the party, were a Cough, a pain in his
Breaft, difficulty of refpiration, and an
Hectick Feaver. The *Pericardium* is likewife fummon'd by *Petr. Salius de cur.
Morb. c.* 7. for an apparent caufe of a
Tabes or *Marcour*, if anywife affected,

a

suppose inflammed, or pustulated. This
may seem strange, that an ignoble part
should bring the whole body in danger; but
when considering its near situation to the
heart, the cause is obvious enough, whence
to derive its Consumptive symptoms.

Some might rather imagine, that the
drying up of the waterish humours contained in the *Pericardium*, (supposed by most
modern Anatomists to be distined for to
moisten and cool the heart) may now and
then impell a man into a Consumption, for
want of which water, the heart dryes away
and shrinks, whereunto the other parts are
obliged to sympathize. But in my opinion
'tis questionable, whether any such waterish
liquor be floating in the *Pericardium*, whilst
a man is yet living; for in Beasts, as Dogs
& Cats, whose breast hath been pierced
alive, to discover, whether the said Membrane the heart is wrapt up in, be moistned
with that kind of serosity, no such thing was
apprehended, in whom notwithstanding
there appeared the same necessity for a
cooler, as in men, whose languishing heart
probably whilst a dying, may seem faintly

to sweat such kind of moist drops into its bag. 2. There have been some, that were born destitute of a *Pericardium*, witness *Columbus lib.* 15. *Anat.* where he recites the Anatomy of a Scholar at *Rome*, whom he found wanting of a *Pericardium*; so *Galen lib.* 7. *cap.* 13. *Administ. Anat.* doth likewise instance a Boy, whose heart lay visible, because the breast bone was part cut out, and the *Pericardium* partly putrefyed.

A dry Consumption may likewise chance upon a *Vomica* or a tumor of humours turn'd into matter and inclosed in a bag, (whereby Authors would have it differenced from an Apostem) in the Lungs, which before it breaks causes a stertour (or noise in the Throat) in breathing, and a very troublesome Asthma.

A Pulmonique Consumption doth sometimes happen upon a *Varix*, or vein swelled in the Lungs, which in length of time doth burst, whence an effusion of blood, and soon after a congestion of purulent matter.

Hippocrates in coac. præd. makes mention of a kind of suppuration, that survenes

Lethargies,

Lethargies, which doth commonly termi‥ nate into a Confumption. *viz. quicunque vero fervantur ex Lethargicis ut plurimum fuppurati fiunt :* thofe that recover of a Lethargy, for the moft part become fuppurated. But *lib.* 1. *de Morb.* he relates five kinds of Pectoral fuppurations more, that tend to the fame period, unlefs according to 15. *Aphor. lib.* 5. they expectorate the matter in 40. dayes. *viz.* Firft, there is a fuppuration of fleam diftilling from the head into the hallow of the breaft. The fecond follows a Pleurifie not expectorated. The third happens upon the burfting of a vein in the breaft. The fourth upon a Phlegmatique Pleurifie. The fifth fucceeds a *varix* in the breaft burfted, or fweating out (*per Diapedefin*) blood.

But thofe that are curious to be further fatisfied touching the manner of Pectoral or Pulmonique fuppurations, let them perufe *Hipp. lib.* 1. *de Morb.* where he doth moft incomparably illuftrate that fubject. Here may be queftioned, *Whether Phleam according to* Hippocrates *his dictate is fuppurable, or difpofed to be converted into*

L 4 *matter ?*

matter ? Pure Phleam certainly is not, but being mixed with other humours is experienced to be fuppurable.

Hippocrates lib. de Glandul. defcribes a Sciatique Confumption (*Tabes coxendica ;*) *Alius morbus oritur ex defluxione capitis per venas in Spinalem Medullam, inde autem in Sacrum os impetum facit, & in coxendicum acetabula, five juncturas deponit, & fi tabem fecerit homo marcefcit; atque hoc modo, contabefcit & vivere non expetit.* i. e. Another Difeafe takes its beginning from a defluxion of the head through the Veins into the Marrow of the Back ; thence forceth to the *os facrum,* and expels (to wit the diftilled humour) into the Hip joynts.

The Lungs do fometimes though very rarely grow faft to the *Pleura* (the skin that lines the breaft within,) whence fuch as are detained with that accident are *Lung-grown :* The fymptoms attending, are a heavy pain in the breaft, a difficulty of refpiration (*breathing,*) faintnefs, *&c.* which continuing do advance their fubjects to a Confumption. This fort of Confumption might be annumerated to an *Afthmatick*

ick Confumption, as *Mercatus* and others
re pleafed to term it, fince the fymptoms
ppear not different from thofe in an
Afthma, faving there is only a Cough want-
ng to make up the train. The caufe of this
Lung-growth is imputed to a fuperficial
anious or ichorous exulceration, whofe
natter being fomewhat glutinous, cleaves to
he forefaid *Pleura*, and dryes up to it,
whereby it's faftned. The truth hereof is
evidenced in the diffected bodies of thofe,
that were Lung-grown, whofe Lungs are
ever found ichorous and mattery near the
place of adhæfion, witnefs the diffected
bodies of *Ferdinand* the Emperour, and
Francis the *French* King, whofe Lungs,
according to the Teftimonies of *Gefner*, and
Holtzach, were not only deprehended faftned to the fides of the breaft, but in a great
part putrefied and fanious. But whether
thofe *filaments* (threds,) that ferve in lieu
of ligaments to tye the Lungs to the *Pleura*,
being fhortned by a ftrain, or imbibition of
humours, may not produce a Confumption,
feems not improbable; an Afthma it's certain they do, and confequently may attract
humours

humours to the Lungs, and prove an accidental caufe of overheating and overdrying the heart, for not expiring the fuliginous fteems, that iffue thence, and not infpiring frefh air fufficient to cool and moiften it. on the other hand, thefe faid filaments being overmuch relaxed, or broken, do induce that accident which may be properly ftiled the Rifing of the Lights. Some other infrequent (*rare*) Confumptions may happen, but fuch as fcarce appear among ten thoufand Confumptives, and therefore fhall forbear their infertion, committing their narrow fearch to Phyficians their proper induftry.

CHAP.

CHAP. XXVIII.

Of the Procatarctick, or external causes of Pulmonique Consumptions.

THose Procatarčticks that required a larger comment, as love, grief, &c. we have difcourfed of in particular Chapt. others that are limitted in a narrower extent of fpeculation, and particularly fuch, as promote *Englifh* Bodies beyond thofe of other Nations into Confumptions, we intend to treat of here.

To begin with thefe latter, it's not improbable the caufes muft be inherent in thofe *non naturals*, whofe quality, and our ufe of them differing from other Nations, tranfport our bodies beyond theirs into extenuations and Marcours.

1. We differ extremely from all others in our dyet. *Flemmings* and *Germans* buy flefh meat by the pound, and eat it by ounces; we buy meat by whole joynts, and eat it by pounds. 2. They

2. They ufually boyl and roaft their meat, until it falls almoft off from the bones , but we love it half raw, with the blood trickling down from it , delicately terming it the Gravy, which in truth looks more like an ichorous or raw bloody matter. 3. Flefh once a week is a variety to their great ones, once a month a delicacy to their Burgers *(Citizen's,)* and once a year a feaft to the rabble, and that at their *Kermiffes* or Fairs only. But their thriving dyet the hogs has taught 'em, *viz.* Cabbage, Turnips, Salates, Butter-milk, Whey, *&c.* Which renders them alike not only in fatnefs, but in manner of humour, witnefs their Brawny Necks, Fat Trype Guts, and grunting hoggifh de-portments. But here on the other hand great and fmall, rabble and all, muft have their Bellyes ftuffed with flefh meat every day, and on Sundayes cramb their guts up to the crop with pudding.

4. Neither is the difference only in the eating part, but drinking, they overwhelming their panch daily with a kind of flat *Scarbier*, or Rotgut; we with a bitter dreggifh fmall liquor, that favours of little elfe

elſe than hops and muddy water. The wine
they ſo much debauch themſelves with, is a
kind of crude dull ſtumd *Burdeaux*; we
with *Canary*. Thus we have parallel'd the
dyets of two Nations, in order to a further
examination of their different effects, rendring thoſe of a ſquabbiſh lardy habit of
body; us of a thinner though more fleſhy
appearance, and ſome who by their ſtronger
natures, exerciſe, or labour, are equally
matcht to digeſt and ſubdue that maſs of
fleſh they daily devour, acquire a double
ſtrength to what thoſe Hermits receive from
their Herbage.

But ſince we experience that ſort of
feeding, doth ſcarce improve our carcaſſes
beyond a lean habit, and the contrary dyet
to ſtuff the hides of our Neighbours with a
large proportion of Greaſe and Tallow,
gives us argument, to impute to it a great
part of the occaſion, that inclines us ſo
much to Conſumptions. Wee'l inſiſt a little
further upon the matter; firſt, touching our
ſo greedy devouring of fleſh, eſpecially
Beef, and Mutton, whereof there is a greater
quantity conſumed in *England*, than in all
Spain,

Spain, *France*, *Holland*, *Zealand*, and *Flanders*, as I can demonstratively make appear to you by this sole instance : you'l grant there are more gloves worn here, then in all *Holland*, *Zealand*, and *Flanders* besides , for from the highest to the lowest they usually go with their hands in their Pockets in the Summer, and in the Winter hold 'em to their Noses to blow 'em warm. Next, we wear out more Shooes here by two thirds than all *France*, where it's universally known, the paysantry goes barefoot, and the middle sort throughout all that Kingdome makes use of Wooden Clogs. Now this considered, that notwithstanding the great number of gloves and shooes worn out here, besides millions of pairs that are transported hence to the *Barbado's*, *Virginia*, and many other Plantations, we abound so much with Hides, Gloves, Sheeps and Neats Leather, that we furnish the better part of all Christendom with them; which is a certain sign there must be an incredible number of Sheep and Oxen killed, whose flesh since we make no forreign Merchandize of, (saving only of their Skins and Hides,)

Hides,) muſt neceſſarily be all conſumed among us. But to declare to you the great miſchiefs (which is my chief buſineſs) this fleſh greedineſs heaps upon us : a Plethory (fulneſs of blood) both *ad vaſa* and *vires*, is the firſt and immediate effect ; the next, a *Plethora ad vaſa* (an over fulneſs of the Veins and Arteries with blood) doth eaſily upon a ſmall commotion or heat of body, fall, or other accidents, burſt a Vein in the Lungs, whereupon commonly follows an Ulcer, and ſoon after a Pulmonique Conſumption.

Moreover, note that a Plethory produced by immoderate eating of fleſh is more impetuous and turgent, and therefore ſo much diſpoſed to burſt a Vein ; whereas any other Plethory engendred of Fiſh, Milk, or Herbs, being leſs turgent, and diluted with wateriſh humours ſeldom ſwells to that height.

The *Plethora ad vires* (a fulneſs of blood, that oppreſſes the ſtrength) is the evident cauſe, that renders us univerſally lean, by ſuppreſſing our ſpirits and hebetating (*dulling*) their vigour, whereby they are not only incapacitated of digeſting the

the alimonious humours into flesh , but of attracting blood to the parts to nourish them ; which defect reduces the body to a leanneſs, and if continued to a Conſump-tion.

Laſtly, know, that fleſh meat being ſo nutritive , and likewiſe hard of digeſture, doth abound with the moſt and worſt dregs of any other kind of meat , eſpecially if not totally digeſted, as ſeldome it is by thoſe that glut down ſuch immeaſurable propor-tions of fleſh. Theſe dregs immediately perfuſe the blood with melancholy , cauſe obſtructions of the Spleen and Liver, and ſtick in the capillar inſertions of the Sto-mach, being ſoon incinerated and calcined into ſuch Salts as we premitted in the pre-ceding Chapter : which after a ſhort inter-lapſe of time produce Coughs, Ptiſicks, and at laſt a Pulmonique Conſumption.

For a further proof hereof wee'l add a dictate or two of *Hippocrates.* lib. de veter. Med. *he ſaith, that Meat eaten in greater quantity than what is convenient , tabefyes* (conſumes) *the body.* And lib. de loc. in homine ; *he ſpeaks thus, If the body conquers the be meat it eats , it flourishes ; but if it be overcome, and yeilds, the body grows lean.*

Now let's pass to the other part of your yet, that so much admired Mistress of your ind Palats, *Canary*, to whose debauchery far greater number of Murders may be nputed, than to the fury of the Sword. That malignant Feavers, Dysenteries, pernicious Consumptions, doth it impell *Engsh* bodies into ? Sack drinkers that somemes have over balasted their panch with nat liquor, do by their beastly return of it resent their Spectators with a view , what most filthy corrosive greenish oyl its conerted into , by the preternatural heat of heir Stomach, which in length of time being congested in some considerable quanity, and floating in a violent stream through he Vessels, is the cause of so many malign eavers , as generally reign here towards he latter end of the Summer. This is the he account of its acute *(quick and violent)* ffects; it's Chronical *(of a longer protralion)* ones are, a vehement drying and nflammation of the bowels and humours, whereby great and obstinate obstructions

M are

are engendred, by drying away and abforbing the fubtiler and more waterifh part of
the humours, and leaving the groffer behind,
which foon turns to an aduft melancholy,
the further effects whereof have been fufficiently declared already.

Neither are the meaner fort of people
deftitute of their *Ambrofia*, who muft needs
every day after Sunfet beftow three pence
out of their groat, in Strong Beer, a liquor
that attributes the better half of its ill qualities to the Hops, being an inland drugg, con-
confifting of an acrimonious fiery nature,
fetting the blood upon the leaft Cacochymy
(*vitious humours*) into an *Orgafmus* (a violent working,) by an ill *ferment* it yeilds to
the Stomach, Liver, and Spleen, which
doth likewife render the humours fiery,
aduft, and melancholique. Small Beer,
though it partakes lefs of the Hops, yet according to their proportion, correfponds
in offenfive and infalubrious (*unwholfome*)
qualities; whence we may obferve, that
Patients in Feavers and many other
diftempers, receive a fenfible prejudice
from that rot-gut, though the quantity o

Hop

ops be lefs; by the forefaid *Orgafmus* it
cites. By this you may judge, fince fmall
er at the beft proves fo unwholfome a
ink, what it doth at worft, perhaps being
ewed with a thick muddy and clayifh wa-
r, which the Brewers covet the rather,
caufe of adding a body or fubftance to the
ink, which the dead remainder and
all quantity of Malt can in no wife con-
ibute to it : now to give a ftrong taft to
is dreggifh liquor, they fling in an incre-
ble deal of Broom, or Hops, whereby
all beer is rendred equal in mifchief to
rong.

The third Endemick caufe, whence we
rive our extenuating difeafes, is the Air,
hich as I have expreffed to you before in
hapt. o. obtains a more particular and
mediate power from its continual com-
erce with our Lungs and Vital fpirits, of
mmitting violence upon them and the
itals. There is none, who hath traverfed
le leaft tract of ground beyond his native
il, but can atteft the ftrange alterations
le Air produces upon bodies, efpecially
difeafed : The Air o'th *Alps* fubjects

M 2   the

the Inhabitants there to diſtillations to their throat, which congeſted do in a ſhort ſpace ſwell into a huge mole ; the *Indian* Air diſpoſes Northern bodies to Dyſenteries; the *Spaniſh* Air engenders the Kings evil; that of *Padua* a blindneſs, where I remember I took notice of ſeveral blind folks, but whether the Air of that place had produced that accident in them, or whether they came from other places thither to be cured by ſtroaking their eye-lids over Saint *Antonio di Padua's* Tomb, by which means great numbers (as they told me) have been reduced to their perfect ſights, I inquired not. The Air at *Rome* is likewiſe very pernicious, eſpecially all the Summer, at which time, as I was informed there , no perſon will hazard to travel towards *Naples*; for fear of incurring that dangerous phrenſie and burning Feaver, which the change of Air unavoidably brings upon them, eſpecially upon thoſe that return from *Naples* to *Rome*, among whom ſcarce one in a hundred eſcapes, though they uſe the extremeſt remedies, as actual cauteries and ſcarifications for their recovery. What calamitou

effeſt

fects the Air of this City wrought upon us he laft year, you may read in my *Difcourfe the Plague.* In fine, thete's no caufe of 1eftioning, but that the Air doth evidently oncur to the production of feveral Difeas, and particularly of this *Englifh* Endeiick; but through what means or difpofion, it's that I am about, to illuftrate to ou. The fituation of this Ifland is fuch, difpofes it to a continual clowdinefs, hich in the fummer renders the Air ooler, and in the Winter warmer. The latter whereout thofe perennal clouds are iifed, is the Sea that cirrounds us, which louds fo attracted, the wefterly winds, lowing three fourths of the year, do continally blow upon us ; in lieu whereof, if aftern winds did perflate our clime more equently, would not only blow away iofe mifty clouds, but exceedingly clarifie id refrefh our Air. Thefe clouds, as they re raifed out of the Sea, fo they ftill parike of the falin (*faltifh*) bodies, they rew up with them thence, which defcendig upon us by degrees, and being perfufed irough the Air, do through their falin acri-

mony

mony corrode our weak Lungs, and with
their thick foggy fubſtance obſtruct the
Bronchia Pulmonum, or Lung-pipes. This
Pulmonique indiſpoſition of the Air, is
very much heightned in great Cities, eſpecially where a great quantity of Sea-coal is
burned, as here in *London,* where the number of Brew-houſes, Cooks, and Smiths
Shops, beſides all other Private houſes,
Brick and Lime Kills about the City, make
ſmoak, that at a diſtance *London* appears in
a morning as if it were drowned in a black
cloud, and all the day after ſmothered with
a ſmoaky fog, the conſequence whereof
proves very offenſive to the Lungs in two
reſpects. 1. By means of thoſe Sulphurous
coal ſmoaks the Lungs are as it were ſtifled
and extremely oppreſſed, whereby they
are forced to inſpire and expire the Air with
difficulty, in compariſon to the facility of
inſpiring and expiring the Air in the Country, as people immediately perceive upon
their change of Air; which difficulty, oppreſſion, and ſtopping muſt needs at length
waſt the Lungs, and weaken them in their
function. 2. Thoſe fuliginous ſmoaks part

confisting of falin corrofive fteems, feem
partake of the nature of *Salt armoniack*,
hereby they gnaw and in time Ulcerate
e tender fubftance and fmall veins of the
ungs. That coal fmoak is of fo corrofive
quality is eafily experienced by thofe, that
e befet with fmoak in a room, whofe eyes
bites and gnaws that it forceth 'em to wa-
r, and by pricking their Throat and Lungs
its them into a dry Cough. Thefe falin
rrofive fteems are very much intended
the addition of thofe, that exhale from
oufes of Office, Piffing places, and other
fty ftinks and fumes great Cities are
er pefter'd with.

Another great caufe of the frequency of
onfumptions among us, and efpecially
out the City, is a continuated defcent
f weak Pulmonique Children from Con-
mptive Parents, who propagate and tranf-
fe their Pulmonique Seminaries to their
hole fubfequent generation; which occa-
ons fo many hundreds to drop hence
very year to the Countrey for frefh air.

Hitherto we have infifted upon thofe
ufes, that effect Confumptions Endemick

mick to this Island; there remains a citation
of such others, as indifferently may produce
that malady in any other Countrey. Immoderate feeding upon Powder'd Beef, Bacon,
Salt Fish, Pickled Meats, Anchiovi, and
debauching with Brandy, Sack, and other
strong Wines and Spirits, do inflame and
acuate the blood, whereby it's capacitated
to corrode the tender veins of the Lungs,
whereupon follows spitting and coughing
up of blood. A fall, (and according to
Hippocrates lib. 2. de Morb.) vehement
exercise or labour, violent vomiting, a
blow upon the breast, calling a lowd, do
oftimes occasion a vein to burst in the
Lungs. Catching cold on the breast, by
going cool in the morning or evening, (as
many do by leaving their Doublets unbut-
toned, or women by running up and down
in their Smock sleeves, or lying naked with
their breast in the night) doth impell the
blood suddenly into the Lung-veins, whereby being overfilled, burst into an effusion
of blood. Those that are naturally destitute,
or have lost their *Uvula*, (palat) are likewise very incident into a rupture of a Lung
vein,

vein, in admitting the cold air, without that previous alteration, the *Columella* (palat) contributed, by hindering the cold air to irrupt suddenly into the Lungs. The eating of a Sea hare is thought to corrode the Lungs by a Specifick property. *Pliny lib.* 7. 2. writes, that there is a certain people in *Æthiopia*, whose sweat precipitates any into a Consumption whom it touches.

Consumptions do frequently arrive upon a sudden suppression of the Hæmorrhoids (*piles,*) witness *Hippocrates* 6. Aph. 12. *If upon curing of Hamorrhoids that have ran long, you do'nt leave one, there is danger of a Dropsie, or Consumption*; because nature was wont to evacuate its burden of vitious Melancholique and Cholerick blood out at those veins, which passage being stopt, it's forced to regurgitate upwards to the Lungs; the like happens upon the stoppage of Womens courses, which if not suddenly look'd to, sets them undoubtedly into a Consumption, Dropsie, or some other dangerous Disease, as *Hippocrates* lib. 2, *de Morb.* also observes. *viz. Si virgo ex suppressione mensium in tabem deveniat,* &c. What constitution of the year is most like to engender Consumptions, *Hip.* tells us: First, for moist Consumptions that survene distillations of sharp putrid fleam, a moist and southerly Autum upon a dry and Northern Summer, is apt to produce them. 3. *Aphor.* 13. Secondly, dry Consumptions generally appear upon a long continuation of hot and dry weather. 2. *Aphor.* 16. *per squalores vero tabes* , &c. The season or time of year for Consumptions is the Autum. 3. *Aphor. Autumno invadunt Febres, Hydropes, tabes,* &c.

CHAP. XXIX.

Of the Signs of a beginning or growing Consumption.

THe surest cure for a Pulmonique Consumption, is to prevent it in those, that are naturally inclined to that evil , or have but lately conceived the Seeds of it, and are just a budding. But because the

pre

reventive part is frequently neglected,
pon hopes of waring it out, or by chang-
ig the air, or for want of knowing the
ate they are in, (which to difcern in the
ommencement is difficult even to Phyfi-
ians themfelves, who are not feldom
iftaken in that point,) the impending
anger whereof requires a mature caution,
fhall delineate fuch natural and adventi-
ous difpofitions, as appear fufpicious.
. To defcend from Phthifical Parents, or
ich as were Pulmonique, that is, affected
ith any kind of trouble in their Lungs, be
t a Cough, difficulty of breathing, Afthma,
r a Pulmonique Confumption, is a great
rgument, fince it's obferved that Confump-
ions prove fo hereditary, and that fome-
imes in a ftrange manner; *viz.* fome
leriving their extenuating Difeafes from
heir Grandfather, though their immediate
Parents did not feem troubled with the
eaft kind of diftemper in their Lungs. The
eafon is, becaufe thofe hereditary feeds
emained dormant in their Parents, and
never were reduced *in actum,* which never
thelefs were transfufed into their Children,

in

in whom they might be raised to growth.
2. Brothers or Sisters taking their passage
through that Disease to their Graves, leave
an ill *omen* to the remainder of their kin.
3. Whom nature hath shaped with a great
head, long neck, narrow breast, and
shoulders sticking out like wings, and a
lean habit of body, seem very much inclined to a Consumption. 4. Such as are subject
to thin sharp Coughs, itching of the Eyes,
a tickling in their Throat, pains of their
Sides, and do not thrive upon a good dyet,
are prepared for a Consumption. 5. To
omit letting blood at certain seasons that
the body is accustomed to, or to escape
bleeding at the Nose, or avoiding blood by
the Hæmorrhoids if usual, or for women
to be obstructed in their courses, argues
danger. 6. Especially at the fall, and in
persons aged from Eighteen to Thirty five
years. 7. To be apt to spit blood oft,
though it distills from the head, or is expressed out of the terminations of veins in
the Throat, signifies a Phthisical inclination,
& is dangerous; because it's a sign, the blood
is sharp and thin, and may upon a small pro-
voci-

vocation vent its fury upon the Lung veins.

8. And laftly, any of the Procatarcktick caufes mentioned in the Chapter preceding, or the beginning of this Treatife, or any other Difeafe, producing a durable leannefs and drynefs of body, with a fhort, dry, or moift Cough, portends an ill confequence, as you may obferve out of *Hipp.* 2. *Aph.* 3. in all Difeafes it's better for the belly to be thick ; on the contrary, when the belly is very thin, and very much confumed it's dangerous.

CHAP. XXX.

Of Signs, Diagnoftick and Prognoftick, of the feveral kinds of fpitting of Blood.

Since fpitting of blood (*haimoptyfis*) doth fo frequently forerun Ulcers in the Lungs, it's requifite I fhould tell you what kind of fpitting of blood forefpeaks danger of a Confumption. Wherefore know,

know, that blood evacuated at the mouth with the spittle, may either distill from the brain, or palat, or be expressed out of the Throat, or Gullet, or forced out of the Stomach, Breast, Mediastinum, Diaphragma, Lungs, or Wind-pipe. Among these, blood forced out of the Lungs gives the worst appearance, and doth seldom vanish without leaving an Ulcer behind it.

Moreover there is a very considerable difference in respect of danger, in blood that issues out of the Lung veins, which are apt to shed their humours upon these four occasions.

1. Upon a rupture or bursting, among the *Greeks* called ϱῆξις.

2. Upon the corrotion of a vein, that is, when it's eaten through by sharp gnawing blood, in *Greek* termed διάβρωσις.

3. A vein gaping or its lips being forced open by a Plethory, is apt to effuse a quantity of blood, in *Greek* called Ἀναστόμωσις.

4. When the Tunicks of the veins are grown thin, and the blood is likewise rendred subtil and piercing, it's apt to sweat
through;

rough, which is nominated a Διαπίδνοις.

This latter is oft cured, and therefore of more hopeful aspect; but the two former or the most part contemn all remedies. he bursting or corrosion of a Vein in the *leura* succeeds these former in a malicious *men.* Any of these bloody sputations be-ig too suddenly cured, oft changes into a agick Scene. The like happens upon xternal applications of restringent me-icines to the breast, or in case internal estrictives be exhibited without dissolvents, o dissolve the crumbs of blood, that usually oncrease out of the extravasated humours, vhich otherwise would occasion a suffoca-ion. A bloody sputation, whether proceed-ng from the Lungs, or Stomach, inti-nates less danger in Women, whose ob-structed courses were the cause of it; be-cause these being carried down do seldom miss a cure of the former, as *Hippocrates* doth likewise aphoristically tell us; *A Woman vomiting blood, her courses breaking forth puts a stop to her vomiting*; but this is to be understood, in case a Vein gapes or is forced open by a Plethory, not if a Vein be bursted or corroded. The

The same reason holds good in men, sur-prized with a sanguin sputation upon a sudden cohibition of their *Hæmorrhoids*, which being recalled do frequently stent the other Symptom ; but if their Hæmor-rhoids have disappeared for a conside-rable time , than such a sputation survening upon it proves more perilous than other-wise.

Spitting of blood is more curable in Plethoricks, and young folks, than in others of a thinner habit of body, and old people, because as *Hippocrates* implyes in 2. Aph. 34. *They are less endangered in Diseases, whose Disease suits with their nature, age, and habit of body, and time, than those whose Disease is in no part agreeable.*

In summa; any kind of spitting of blood imports a very discriminous state, unless it happens as I said before upon the gaping of a Vein, or being opened, (but not bursted or corroded) by a Plethory, in which case it's a great help to nature, being over burden'd with blood ; and it usually stops of it self. Thus I have known several women vom't up great quantities of blood, possibly a

pint

oint or two, without any prejudice. Some I have heard of, that have coughed up a quantity not much lefs, no kind of detriment following upon it. A Vein burfted or corroded in the Lungs, is look'd upon to be for the moft part incurable (though fome do efcape,) becaufe of the continual motion and Coughing of the Lungs, taring the gap wider, and hindering the conglutination and cicatrization of the vein; befides their remote diftance from the Stomach, the vertues of Medicines, being quite fpent before they can arrive thither. Spitting of blood being complicated with other chronical Difeafes, as great obftructions of the Bowels, Afthma, &c. is rendred lefs capable of cure than otherwife. A *varix* or a fweld vein in the Lungs doth oft a good while after burft out into a fudden fpitting of blood, the patient not dreaming of the leaft Difeafe his body fhould be fubjected to; for the Lungs being infenfible within, cannot advert him of any tumour or fwelling. This accident ufually happens, when a man hath had a fall, or bruife upon his breaft, whereby the groffer part of the

N

blood

blood was suddenly impelled into a Vein of the Lungs, where it causes that swelling, which possibly may burst a month or six weeks after, for want of taking something at the beginning to dissolve the impulsed blood.

A broken Vein conglutinated, or a corroded one cicatrized, is very apt upon a small irritation, as a cough, vomit, fall, &c. to burst again, or return to an Ulcer, because the cicatrize, or agglutination is performed by a dissolvable, or sometime friable kind of humour, that's easily colliquated, or rent asunder by the continual motion of the Lungs, and especially if render'd violent by a Cough, or other accident. Wherefore persons that have been so indisposed, ought to refrain from taking Vomits, or moving their bodies violently; & timely to remedy any kind of Cough, or other Pulmonique Diseases.

We have given you a large comment of the Prognosticks of spitting blood ; the remainder of this Chapter wee'l imploy in the Diagnosticks. Blood that's evacuated from the Lungs is forced up with a Cough without

without any pain, and if a Lung-vein be burſted, generally at the firſt guſh a great quantity is cough'd up, which afterwards comes up in ſmaller proportions.

The blood that's evacuated at firſt, appears thin, pure, and florid, with a little yellowiſh froth upon it; that which is afterwards evacuated, ſhews paler, and watered, with a few bubles on it; at laſt it's expectorated mixt with fleam. That which ſweats through the veins, comes up diſuted (*pale and watered*) in ſmall quantities mixt with fleam, ſpittle, or ſome of the *ſerum* of the blood.

If a Lung Vein be corroded, the blood at firſt comes up in a ſmaller quantity; afterwards in fuller ſtreams. Phyſicians do vary much in the colour of Pulmonique blood that's evacuated, ſome will have it a purple, others a florid, yellow, or natural red. As to that, Lung-blood generally appears ſomewhat lighter than a natural red, becauſe its conceived to be rendred more aereous by the Lungs. Nevertheleſs it varies according to the conſtitution of bodies; for in ſome it may be purple, in others yellow, or red. Another difpute that's moved among Authors is, whether Lung-blood is alwayes evacuated with a Scum or froth upon it, according to *Hippoc.* 5. Aph. 13. *Thofe that fpit out frothy blood with coughing, it comes from the Lungs.* For to decide this controverfie; you muft note, there is a fourfold fubftance concurring to the conftitution of the Lungs.

1. The Grifly fubftance of the Lung-pipes.

2. The tough fubftance of the Ligaments, that tye the great Veffels to the Lungs, and joyn the pipes together.

3. The *Parenchyma* or flefh of the Lungs.

4. That which the fmall veins and arteries confift of. This confidered, obferve that the blood that's evacuated out of the pores of the corroded *Parenc.* of the Lungs, is ever frothy, becaufe it's forced through a number of fmall holes or pores in the Lungs, whereby it's rarefyed and rendred frothy. But the blood that's caft out of the greater Veffels is not alwayes thoroughly frothy, but only a top, which is caufed by it's being mingled with the Air in the coughing it up; and for
that

:hat reafon blood that's vomited up, may
ilfo appear frothy, as *Hippocrates lib. de
Coacis,* tells us, thofe *that fpit up* (vomit
up) *frothy blood, and are troubled with their
right fide*) *they fpit it from the Liver, and
commonly dye.* Thus likewife we fee that
blood evacuated in a *Dyfentery* is frothy
a top. So *Avicen* doth witnefs, the blood
to be frothy, that's propel'd out of a Vein
of the Breaft; and *Paulus* writes the blood
out of the Throat to be frothy. Laft of all
you muft diftinguifh between pure blood,
which ufually is expectorated lefs frothy,
than that which is mixt with windy fleam
and melancholy, or only windinefs.

This fimple bloody fputation of the
Lungs is differenced from that, which con-
comitates a pleurifie, or a *Peripneumonia*
(inflammation of the Lungs;) becaufe thefe
two latter are ever painful, to wit a pleurifie is attended with a ftitch, the other
with a heavy pain of the breaft, befides
other Diagnoftick fymptoms; whereas a
fimple blood fpitting arrives without any
pain or feaver. Blood that's caft out of the
throat or wind-pipe, is fpit out with a

hawking

hawking, or a small cough, and that in small quantities or streaks ; that out of the Gums is spit out without hawking, coughing, or vomiting ; that out of the breast is expelled with a difficult cough, and shews lived and full of crumbs ; but blood that distills from the head, since it may be ejected by cough, vomit, hawking, or spiting, may easily delude both Patient and Physician, unless there be a narrow inspection made, for sometimes a small vein bursting in the head will trickle down (but with a tickling in the Throat) in great streams into the wind-pipe or stomach, whence it's returned by cough, or vomit; the usual way to find out the spring of this flood, is to cause the Patient to gargle twice or thrice a sharp *Oxycrate*, which will either stop the cough, or appear with a deep tincture.

Another way for tryal is, that the Patient is to hold his mouth full of water, and blow his Nose hard, by which means if there be a vein burst in the head, some blood will come forth at the Nostrils. Moreover the Physician is to enquire into the

the Procatarctick caufes, whether the party be troubled with a Head-ach, or hath had a fall, or taken cold, and is enrheumed, or the face be high colour'd.

Blood that's ejected by vomit, no doubt but comes out of the Stomach-veins, but whether it be blood that's deftined for its nourifhment, or whether fent from the Spleen or Liver, & effufed into the Stomach through the *Splenick* branch, or *Gaftrick* vein, is alfo nicely fearch'd into by Practick Authors.

If the evacuated blood be florid it's Stomach-blood, if black and in great quantity, it's Splenetick; if red and copious, it's Hepatick. Moreover, if the blood be Splenetick, figns appear of an affected Spleen; if Hepatick, of the Liver.

CHAP

CHAP. XXXI.

*Of the Diagnostick signs of a confirm'd
Consumption of the Lungs.*

YOu must appeal to your memory to
have read in the foregoing part of this
Treatise the distinction of Proper and Improper Consumptions; this latter we
have dissected into its several kinds, among
which I am only to tell you, that an Improper Pulmonique Consumption is deciphered with nothing but a kind of a Pulmonique Disease, be it a Cough, *Dyspnæa,
Asthma,* &c. and a discernable wasting of
the flesh, protracted to some continuance,
which doth certainly menace the sudden
consequence of a Proper Ulcerous Pulmonique Consumption.

As to the evidencing a confirm'd Consumption of the Lungs, the signs are these.

1. There is an old Cough, contracted
possibly at the latter end of the fall, or in
the

the winter, or the firſt approch of the Spring, and continuing for three, ſix, or nine months, without ſpitting blood the whole time.

2. Obſerve that ſuch a cough. that proves ſo durable, doth not alwayes continue at the ſame ſtand, but is far more urgent ſometimes than otherſome, and ſomewhiles again returns to that remiſſion, that it ſeems to be quite gone, until the patient relapſes of his own accord, without any provocation of an external cauſe or errour, into the ſame or rather worſe ſtate than before.

3. The matter expectorated is thick, tough, glewy, frothy, uneven, bubbly, graiſh; or thin, liquid, crude; or thin and mixt with thick, clotty, blewiſh, yellow, greeniſh or blackiſh fleam, or ſtreaks only.

4. A difficulty of breathing, with a kind of a whieſing noiſe.

5. Violent ſtitches up and down the breaſt, and back, below the ſhoulders, which for a while are moveable; afterwards fix either under the ſhoulders or paps, which then give a ſtrong preſumption of a confirm'd *Phthiſis*.   6. The

6. The face looks deadifh, and livid, with a dark blewifh or brown circle about the under eyelids, the eyes appear hollow, flat, and fhrunk, without their natural glofs.

7. All this while the appetit is wanting, and is bent to nothing more than to a draught of ftale ftrong Beer, though that be as bad as rots-bane for 'em: and this is a very ufual attendant.

8. The body is fometimes loofe, and fometimes bound; or in fome it's generally loofe, and in others contrary.

9. They fleep unquietly, and difturbed with fiery or melancholique dreams, and feel hot and glowing at their waking, being likewife much difpofed to fweat about their breaft, neck, and head. Their limbs do oft feel fore and weary. For the moft part they are drowfy and lumpifh all day. By this time an Hectick Feaver begins to fhew it felf, by a quick, foft, low, and unequal pulfe; a fmall glowing of the palms of the hands and feet after meat, &c.

This is the firft degree of a confirm'd Pulmonique Confumption, from which the

the second degree differs in the intension of the forementioned Symptoms; namely,

1. The Cough sounds more hollow and deep; continues longer before any matter is brought up; and is more urgent in the night than the day.

2. The humours or fleam that are expectorated, are turn'd into a thick matter (*pus.*)

3. The body is consumed to nothing but skin and bones; the flesh of the Muscels being withered into dry tough strings, the skin feeling rough and dry like Leather : And the face changed into an *Hippocratean visage*, otherwise called *a Mortiferous face*, and deciphered 1. *progn.* 7. viz. *a sharp Nose; hollow Eyes; the Temples fallen and retch'd; the Ears cold and contracted, and their fibres turn'd; the skin about the forehead hard, retch'd, and shrunk; the colour of the Face is Greenish or Blackish.*

4. At this degree the Legs and Belly usually swell, and sometimes burst out at the toes into a water.

5. The appetit is quite lost.

6. A

6. A senfible Hectick Feaver, ever grow-ing higher in the night then in the day, be-caufe the cold of the night ftops the pores; it's known by a quick, hard, low, uneven in motion and fortitude, Acre or ftinging Pulfe, and a glowing heat of their body an hour or two after Victuals.

7. It's ordinary for Confumptives in this degreeto entertain their vifiters with ftrange rambling difcourfes, of their intent of go-ing here and there, or doing this and that, as if they did in no wife expect to change their dwellings into a grave.

8. They are extremely fretful and pee-vifh; never well at reft, but always calling for this or that, or changing their feats or pofture of lying or fitting.

9. They are incident to Convulfions in their Necks, and Gripes in their Bellies.

10. They are very fubject to *Nocturnal pollutions* (or evacuations of the Sperm without Phanfie,) the reafon whereof *Ariftotle* gives 5. *Probl.* 53, becaufe fharp colliquations falling to the fpermatick parts, excite the excretive faculty,

11. *Ariftotle* among his Problems doth like-

likewife write, that Confumptives are very apt to breed Lice, which probably are engendred out of their clammy fweat, by a putredinal heat that attends them.

12. Their Cheeks appear oft of a rofie red colour, efpecially after meat.

13. At laft they fpit out peices of their Lungs, it may be fmall grifly bits, that are eaten off from the Lung pipes, or fmall light uneven pieces of fpungy flefh.

14. If you defire a particular remarque whereby to know which of the parts are moft apt to confume firft, that fo you may be forewarned in time, I'le refolve you : A Confumption is no where fo vifible as at the fingers ends, whofe flefh commonly fhrinks before any other part of the body, and that for two reafons. 1. Becaufe it's the fineft, tendereft, and moft delicate kind of flefh, confifting of a moft exact temperature, whereby it's the better difpofed for the touch, no part of the body feeling fo exactly; which tender confiftence renders it the more colliquable and confumptive.

2. Becaufe the heat of the body reflecting at the fingers ends, redoubles, and is more intenfe

intenſe than in any other part, as doth more evidently appear in Feavers.

The laſt and third degree foretell the nearneſs of their *fate*, which for the moſt part follows within three or four dayes upon the appearance of theſe ſigns, which *Hippocrates* doth orderly digeſt in 5 *Aphor.* 14. and 7. *Aphor.* 72. *After the evacuating of blood upwards follow a Tabes, (an exquiſite Conſumption,) and evacuation of matter upwards; after a Tabes a defluxion from the head; after a defluxion a looſneſs and a ſtoppage of the expectoration; and after the ſtoppage, death.* To be more particular. 1. There is a looſneſs, whereby the matter that ſhould be evacuated upwards by Cough, is drawn downwards, or rather fixt in the Lungs; not only ſo, but the Spirits, that ſhould actuate the Lungs in the expectoration, are conſumed, diſperſed, and drawn downwards, whereby the Lungs are rendred unable of Coughing up the purulent matter, which remaining cauſes a ſtoppage, that doth ſuddenly choak the heart. 2. A ſhedding of the hair is another fatal ſign, hapning only at laſt, when the body is quite

quite dryed up, and contains not fo much excrementitious moifture, as to nourifh the hair, read 5. *Aphor.* 12. *Quibuscunque tabidis capilli fluunt,* &c. 3. A ftinking breath, a fign the purulent matter is affeted with the worft degree of putrefaction, the immediate effect whereof is a *fator* or ftink. 4. The Nails of the Fingers and Toes bending, or turning crooked like the claws of a Beaft. This arrives becaufe the flefh underneath is confumed, whereupon they are dryed into a crooked round fhape like horns, that bend crooked by being over dryed by lying in the Sun, or before the Fire. 4. Frequent fweats, efpecially on their breaft. 5. *Rhafes lib.* 4. *Con.* writes, that Confumptives, when they are near death, grow light headed. This fign holds true in fome, but not in others, many dying with their perfect underftanding and memory. Yet this is frequent, that their fight grows dimme, and therefore can not fee at that diftance they could before, which makes them oft imagine they fee ftrange things, which they don't. Their hearing is alfo grown very dull upon a fudden

den

den; for otherwife Confumptives in the firft and fecond degree have a very fharp hearing. 6. their voice is very hoarfe. 7. The fpittle of Confumptives being powred upon burning coals, ftinks very ftrong. 5. *Aphor.* 11. *Cum tabi implicitis, quod tuffiendo excluditur fputum, graviter oleat, dum carbonibus ardentibus infunditur, capillique defluant, funeftum.* 8. they fetch their breath at laft very eafily, yet not without the fenfe of a great clogg at their Stomach; and a whiefing or whiffling in their Windpipe. 9. Their Pulfe is intermittent every fixth or eighth Pulfation, in others it's *caprizans, myurus,* or *formicans.* 10. Their Feet and Legs dye firft; which commonly are cold and dead a quarter of an hour or more before the other parts.

Thus we have delineated the whole Hiftory of a Confumption, that abfolves its courfe without fpitting of blood. There remains only an obfervation or two upon that, which is attended with a bloody fputation, which either happens at the beginning, whereupon neceffarily follows the fpitting of matter, according to that *Apho-rifm*

rifm, *Poft fanguinis fputum, puris fpu-tum*, &c. Whether the matter expectorated be fleam, or *pus (matter that's bred in an Ulcer)*is known by ftirring it with a ftick ; if it be fleam, it will cleave and ftick ; if *pus*, it will divide and feparate ; or thus, being dropt into a Bazon of Salt-water, if it defcends to the bottom in a grayifh pow-der like flower, it's purulent matter ; if it fwims, its's fleam ; if it partly fwims and partly finks, it's a mixt fubftance : If the Ulcer in the Lungs be deep in the *Parenchy-ma*, it's difcovered by a hard Cough ; and if almoft reaching to the *Ambient Mem-brane*, then there is a fore kind of pain with a hard cough ; but if the cough be painful and the matter comes up eafie, it's a fign the Ulcer is in the wind-pipe, as the expe-ctorated cartilaginous particles do further declare. The Patient having for a while cough'd up purulent matter, is ever and anon upon a fit of coughing, fretting, or anger, or any other commotion of hu-mours apt to expectorate fmall quantities of diluted blood with fleam.

O   Wee'l

Wee'l put an Epilogue to this Chapter, inferting only the figns of matter expectorated through the Lungs from a fuppuration of the breaft. The proper figns of a fuppuration are comprehenfively mentioned by *Hippocrates lib. de coac. prænot.* 49. *Those that are grown fuppurated efpecially upon a Pleurifie, and Peripneumonia, (which is alfo to be fuppofed upon a Squinfie, the fuppuration whereof is more dangerous than any other) are troubled with fmall heats in the day, but violent in the night, and do fpit nothing out, that is worth taking notice of ; they fweat about the neck and fhoulders, and their eyes grow hollow; and their cheeks are red ; but the extremities of their fingers are worfe hot and rough. Their Nails are turn'd crooked, and grow cold; and there arife tumours about their legs, and pufstules about their bodies; they have an averfion from Victuals.* Befides thefe, 1. there preceded a diftillation of Rheum from their head, or a Pleurifie, Squinfie, or Inflammation of the Lungs. 2. A Feaver, according to 2. *Aphor.* 47. *Whil matter is engendring, pains and feaver arife*

arife, &c. 3. Beating or aking pains.
4. Great fhiverings and difficulty of breathing, near the time of the tumour breaking;
which being broke, the Feaver and pains
abate, and the matter (if not expectorated)
is propell'd into the capacity of the breaft,
where upon the Patients ftirring or turning
himfelf abed from one fide to another, it
makes a fluctuating kind of noife, like the
rumbling of water in a Cask. After a while
it corrodes the ambient membrane of the
Lungs, and is expectorated with a hard
deep or hollow cough.

CHAP. XXXII.

*Of the Prognofticks of a Pulmoniqne
Confumption.*

AS the kinds of Pulmonique Confumptions are various, fo are their Prognofticks, wherefore we muft inftance thefe
latter in the connumeration of the former.
Firft, touching the Sex, and Ages a Con-

O 2   fumptio

fumption is harbour'd in. Children *cæteris paribus* are more frequently cured than thofe of riper years; next Women, who as they are lefs difpofed to the furprize of Confumptions, by reafon of their courfes carrying thofe acrimonious humours away, before they can attain to make any head; fo for the fame reafon, their cure, when at any time illapfed into that Difeafe, is eafier performed than in men; among whom old men that are Confumptive, are the leaft capable of help, becaufe naturally they abound fo much with falt fleam, that heightens and irritates the continent caufe of their malady. Before we deviate from this particular of the Sex, take in this obfervation; that women whilft a breeding, are now and then allarum'd at the fecond month with Confumptive fymptoms, that are caufed through the return of their courfes (being intercepted) to their Lungs.

Among thefe many dye tabefyed before the full expiration of their time; others that have the good fortune of mifcarrying, or being delivered, efcape by means of their floods, revelling the humours from their Lungs.

Lungs. Some again through their straining, pressing, impatient cryes, and commotion of their bodies, at the time of their labour, do sometimes break a vein in their Lungs or Breast, or cause a *varix*, or corrosion of a Vein, whereupon a Consumption following speaks a very hazardous case : or if a Consumption surprizes a Childbed woman, that hath not been well laid, or hath not been well purged after delivery, foretells an equal danger.

The procatarctick causes render the Disease more or less curable : a Consumption of grief, as it moves more flowly than others, so its malign effects are impressed with a more certain and irresistable force; wherefore unless prevented in the bud, takes an ineradicable root. Next hereunto for obstinacy of cure are an *Hypochondriack, Amorous,* and a *Studious* Consumption. As for a *Cachettick* and *Aguish* Consumption they admit usually of an easier cure than others. A *Poysonous, Ulcerous, Renal, Dorsal, Verminous, Bewitch'd, Dolorous, Apostematick,* and *Pockie* Consumptions are more or less curable, or incurable, ac-

cord-

cording to the Age, Sex, Climat, Seaſon of the year, Habit, Temperament, Part affected, Duration, and other ill ſymptoms attending the Diſeaſe.

Having but curſorily propoſed to you a declaration of the preſages of Baſtard Conſumptions, wee'l imploy the more time and paper in relating the Prognoſtick ſigns of Pulmonique Conſumptions, according to the ſeveral degrees obſerved in the preceding Chapter.

A Conſumption of the Lungs in the beginning is very curable, but herein differs from all other curable Diſeaſes, that it's not to be worn away by change of dyet, or moderate exerciſe of body, or a cheerful ſpirit, whereby many other maladies have been diſlodged; but in ſtead of being demulced by counterpoiſing preſervatives of the Patient, goes on its way, until it hath made an abſolute conqueſt of the body; and notwithſtanding though remedies be uſed at its firſt appearance, unleſs they are preſcribed by a dexterous hand, ſo as to hit the humour of the Diſeaſe, and temperament o the Patient, like a Cancer is rather irritate

an

nd eats deeper into the parts. So that Confumptives, though their cafe appears not with fo difcriminous an afpect, ought not only to be follicitous for remedies againft their evil, but to be affured of their skill that apply 'em; for a fault committed in the cure at firft, admits of no appeal afterwards.

The firft degree of a Pulmonique Confumption implyes a difficult and long cure; and may eafily upon neglect of the patient, or ufage of improper Medicines be render'd incurable.

The fecond degree is formidable; and but few of this rank recover, and many more are turn'd over into the Empiricks pit. However wee'l add fome notes out of *Hippocrates* to difcern the curables from the incurables. 1. Their fpittle muft be tryed, if it ftinks being poured upon the coals; or finks as it's caft into a Bafon of falt water; or being fpit upon the ground, if it fhews with round clear fpecks like glafs fpectacles, fignifies a defperate and irrecoverable condition. The like prefage read in a gray, blew, yellow, green, black, mixt, and uneven fpittle. Take a furvey of

O 4 *Aret*

Aret. lib. de fig. & cauf. Morb. diut. cap. 8.
If on the other hand the fpittle appears firft
fanious, afterwards mattery, white, fmooth,
even, and without ftink, there's fome hopes.
2. If the Patient be free from a putrid
Feaver, that increafes in the night, is another hopeful fign. 3. They muft be free
from drought, which confirms the abfenfe
of a putrid Feaver, otherwayes frequently
affecting Confumptives in the beginning
and firft degree. 4. The flood of humours,
that ufed to diftill into the Lungs, muft be
diverted (or rather derivated) through the
Noftrils. 5. It's alfo fuppofed, the party
be not reduced to the greateft extenuation.
6. His ordure muft be rather hard, than
foft, for a loofenefs is generally very pre-
judicial. 7. It's required the Party fhould
have a fquare, flefhy, and hairy breaft, and
not very bony, which fignifies a competent
ftrength of nature in the Patient. If the
contrary figns appear, you muft look for
nothing but death. The cafe is the fame
with thofe who feel a great oppreffion upon
their breaft, fpeak hoarfe, and feem to
have a ftiff neck, (or at leaft is not very
flexible,

flexible,) and the joynts and knuckles of their Fingers fhew big, and their bones fmall : Add hereunto the fymptoms of the third degree, which bring death along with them.

You are alfo to make diftinction of the part affected; for an Ulcer of the breaft is of a lefs difficult cure than one in the wind-pipe, and that in the veffels of the Lungs worfe than it; but an Ulcer in the fubftance of the Lungs is the moft deplorable of any, which the Univerfity of Phyficians declare abfolutely incurable, though *Hippocrates* feems to affert fome curable, namely in whom the feven forementioned conditions are deprehended. Which fentiment we find likewife confirm'd by the experience of feveral reputed Authours; *Cardan* in his Treatife *de Cur. Admirand.* No. 2. 4. 5. 6. 7. 10. recites many Confumptives by his care and skill perfectly reftored; among which number were feveral of the fecond and third degree; but I doubt he quack't a little fometimes : however *Eraftus* exceeds him in afferting cures much more incredible. Saith he, in his *Difp. Paracelf.* part. 1.

pag.

pag. 210. *I'le tell you some thing, that's*
hard to be believed : God hath restored some
Consumptives, that made use of my help,
who it was clearly apparent, scarce beheld
the half of their Lungs.   And in another
place he vaunts to have cured many Consumptives in the beginning, and some that
were absolutely desperate.   *Ingrassias in*
Consil. pro sist. pett. Franc. Arcæus de febr.
cap. 8. *Valleriola* lib. 2. *Observ.* 3. *lib.* 3.
Obs. 6. *& lib.* 5. *Obs.* 5. 6. *Hælidæus. lib.* 3.
Consl. 7. *Beniven. de Abl. c.* 44. *Forest.*
lib. 16. *Obs.* 58. *Crato Consl.* 152. *Poterius*
cent. 3. *cap.* 19, 20, 21. and among the
Ancients *Avicen. lib.* 3. *Sen.* 10. *Tract.* 5.
cap. 5. *Rases* 4. *cont. Valesc. de taranta*
lib. 3. *cap.* 2. *Abynzoar. lib.* 1. *Theysir.*
tract. 11. *cap.* 2. *Mesues cap. de Phthisi,*
besides many others, do bring in perfect
cures of Consumptives of all degrees ; but
questionless performed with great difficulty, because of the continual motion and
coughing of the Lungs, (thereby taring the
Ulcer wider) and their remote distance ;
and at last the Ulcer is only covered with a
limber *callus* , that easily falls off, upon
                                              any

ay commotion of body, cough, or cold
aken in the breaft, and fo forceth patients
into an incurable ftate.

An Hereditary Confumption, likewife
one that's engendred by malign arfenical
fumes under ground (whereunto thofe that
dig in Mines and Coal pits are much fubjected) are incapable of any fort of cure.

A fpitting of blood that happens upon
the burfting of a Lung-Vein, unlefs it be
ftopped or conglutinated in three or four
dayes at fartheft, either occafions a
Phlegmone or inflammation of the Lungs,
which fuppurating turns to an incurable
Ulcer, and a Proper Confumption; or by
evacuating an infupportable meafure of
blood kills the Patient by inducing a *Syncope* (Swoun;) or fuffocates him by coagu-
lating in the Lung-pipes.

An Ulcer in the left lobes is more perilous than in the right, becaufe it's nearer to
the heart. The fame reafon makes a fuppuration contained on the right fide of the
Mediaftinum more dangerous than on the
left.

A

A Confumption enfuing upon a fpieting of blood is of quicker termination, than one that's occafioned by an Ulcerous difpofition of the Lungs, and fomented by falin diftillations from the brain, which may be protracted to fome years. *Avicen* and *Erotian* write of a Woman that was Confumptive three and twenty years together. *Jul. Alexandrinus* and *Mat. de Grad. cap.* 54. *com. in* 9. *lib. Rafis* fpeak of another woman that lived Confumptive eight and twenty years. *Foreftus* knew another woman that ftrove eight years with a Confumption. Neither is this cafe very rare in this City, there being many, I can atteft of, that have been lingring for many years, though affected with a Chronical cough, difficulty of refpiration, and an extreme lean habit of body. The reafon of this prorogation is imputed to a certain abforbing falin diftillation, which being imbibed by the Lungs, is not fo corrofive as to gnaw Ulcers into the Lungs, but doth only abforb their nutriment, and infenfibly diminifh their *Parenchyma*, whereunto the whole body fympathizing, is alfo infenfibly emaciated. But
that

that which is far rarer is, that Ulcerous
Confumptions of the Lungs fhould extend
to fo long fpace, as *Arculanus* reports of
two that fpitted matter four years together.

   We have referved this infertion touching
the Prognofticks of this Difeafe by the Urin
for the Epilogue of the Chapter, which
ufually is various throughout the whole
courfe of the Difeafe: in the firft degree it's
thick and turbid, with a pretty deal of fetling; at the fecond it appears thin and obfcure without any fediment, or very little,
and of a pale ftraw colour, and a greenifh
circle a top;though in fome I have obferved
it bloody and obfcure, like water, where
raw flefh hath been wafhed in; in others it's
thin and blackifh. At laft it's evacuated
clear like water, and in a fmall quantity;
yet this is not Univerfal.

CHAP.

CHAP. XXXIII.

The Therapeutick for Consumptions.

IT's a double misery to be pursued by a lingring Disease, whose nature and cause are disguised under a cloud of various symptoms, which if otherwise appeared in a more visible dress, would it self betray what remedies were most likely to remove it : since therefore Consumptions assault us in that obscure manner, I have engaged my study and industry, to procure you in the preceding discourse a most ample Narrative of that malady, comprizing the total of all observations thereunto relating, that so that intestine enemy being discovered might with more certainty be aggressed, according to the implicit meaning of that trite saying, *a Disease once known is half cured.* So that the greater pains I have taken in the speculative will very much alleviate me in describing the Practick or Therapeutick, whose office is distributed into three parts, *viz.* the *Conservative,*

Pre-

Preſervative, and *Curative*. The *Conſervative* part in this Treatiſe is chiefly concerned in preſerving a healthful body in the ſame ſtate againſt all external cauſes, that may diſpoſe or force it into a Conſumption; Such are the ſix *non naturals*, viz. *a Conſumptive Air*, *and emaciating Dyet*, *Motion* and *Reſt*, the *Excretions* and *Retentions*, *Sleep* and *Reſtleſſeneſs*, and the *Paſſions of the mind*.

If you find your ſelf obliged to live in a Conſumptive Air as this of *London*, make choice of the more open, high, dry, and gravelly part of it, where the houſes are built Eaſt and Weſt, ſhunning thoſe cloſe, low, naſty, dirty and ſtinking Allies, and Lanes near the *Thames* ſide, where the Air being damp, and repleniſh'd with putrid and ſtinking vapours, is pen'd up, and obſtructed from being ventilated by the winds, or its one free motion. 2. Once a day at leaſt take a walk in the Fields, to refreſh your ſelf with the open Air, which inſpired freſh doth exceedingly recreate the Lungs, Heart, and the Vital ſpirits, and through its tenuity opens the Lung-pipes, and purges

purges them from all thofe thick footy fteems; Moreover, opens all the pores of the body, and gives vent to thofe excrementious evaporations. 3. Retreat fome times into the Country for a day, three or four to feaft your Lungs with that pure clear air, and to purge them from the fmoak of *London*.

Touching your dyet obferve thefe Rules: 1. Never tye your felf to a conftant dyet, as alwayes to eat meats of eafie digefture, as Veal, Pullets, Sweatbreads, &c. refufing this becaufe it's obftructive, as Beef, Venifon, Bacon, &c. or that becaufe hard of digefture as Pork, Geefe, Ducks, hard Cheefe, Bifcuit, &c. or becaufe it's loofening, as Cabbage, Spinage, &c. or raw and windy as Salats, Cherries, Apples, &c. for if every objection againft this, or that fort of meat, will caufe you to refrain, than you muft refolve to live without Victuals, there being no meat in the world, but what may be excepted againft, in faying this is windy, and that is ftopping, &c.

Neither would I have you to be too ftrict in the quantity of your meals; as alwayes

I

to leave off with an appetite, or to forbear
eating Suppers upon the account, that it
may hinder your reft.

Neither is't overwholſome to feed con-
ſtantly upon fleſh, refuſing fiſh, and other
victuals, as peaſe, beans, *&c.* arguing as
ſome ſimply do, that fleſh breeds fleſh.

Likewiſe for drink ; be not ſo ſcrupu-
lous as to refuſe a glaſs of Wine, upon
pretence that it's inflaming, neither eſtrange
your ſelf from ſmall Beer, as ſome Drunkards do, fearing it will bring 'em into a
Dropſie. But on the contrary keep a looſe
dyet, feed ſometimes upon fiſh, peaſe,
ſalats, ſpoon meat ; other times upon fleſh,
eggs, roaſt, boyl'd or fryed meats. Sometimes eat liberally, othertimes ſparingly ;
drink ſometimes ſmall beer, ſometimes
ſtrong, or wine. Sometimes eat Suppers,
othertimes faſt.

However miſtake me not, I tell you once
ore, that a looſe and inconſtant dyet is the
moſt wholſome to thoſe that are healthful,
according to that *adage, Sanis omnia ſana.*
The arguments for this aſſertion are theſe.
1. God Almighty having created that variety

riety of creatures for mans food, we are not to doubt but they are wholsome, because he hath created them for our sustentation; not our destruction. 2. We may observe in the new Testament, that Christ sometimes fed upon fish, othertimes upon flesh; sometimes drank water, somtimes wine; somtimes he prayed and fed sparingly, othertimes frequented feasts, where he met with varieties. And in the Old Testament the Patriarchs fed promiscuously upon herbs, most sorts of flesh and fish, whom we cannot question but were most skilful in dyets, as their long protracted ages attested. 4. If God had thought flesh meat only best for us, he would never have provided all these other creatures, as fish, and herbs, for mans food (all things being created for him,) unless necessary to be eaten with other Victuals; for flesh or fish single woul otherwise have been sufficient; besides *God and Nature do nothing in vain.* 5. Th eagerness of the appetite is a sign of th proneness and readiness of the Spirits i and about the Stomach to digest; but t appetite being generally more eager aft

varie

variety of meats, it's a fign the fpirits are more prone and ready to digeft them. On the other hand, one being tyed to a fingle and conftant difh; his Stomach doth not much long for Dinner or Supper; and as he eats without appetite, fo he digefts it heavily, which muft neceffarily contract crudities and ill humours. 6. The fpirits of the Stomach growing familiar with the Victuals daily ingefted, do not only digeft them imperfectly, but are flug in their excretive faculty in evacuating the excrementitious humours; which is more apparent in this inftance, a man that doth feed upon one difh at a Meal, fhall nothing near evacuate (or in plain *Englifh*, go to ftool) fo quick or readily as one that dines upon two or more; becaufe there is generally a contrariety between feveral meats, which doth not only augment the fermentation in the Stomach, but excites and ftirs the digefting fpirits, & afterwards prompts them to a ready evacuation. Laftly, one that dyets upon variety, hath this convenience, that what's deficient in one Meal is fupplyed by another, or what is faulty in one, is corrected

P 2 by

by the other; if one day you have engendred obstructions by eating too much pudding, rice, bread, &c. eat the more Spoon
meat next day, and so you are right again;
or if you have drank too much small beer at
dinner, and thereby oppressed your Stomach
with crudities, drink wine at supper. Or
if you have exceeded in quantity at one
time, eat or drink less at another. *In summa*,
accustome your self to no kind of victuals
or drink, neither to time or quantity; but
follow these Rules. 1. Eat flesh meat four
or five times a week; and fish twice or
thrice, whereby you'l qualify the dryer and
overstrong juice of flesh, by tempering it
with the moister and weaker of the fish.

2. Never make a meal of flesh alone,
but have some other meat with it of less
nutriture, as in the Summer, Pease, Beans,
Artichoaks, Salats, &c. in the Winter
Butter'd Wheat, Milk Pottage, Broaths,
or *Souppes*. 3. A small excess committed
now and then is no wise hurtful, through
means whereof the supervacaneous humours
are stirred, and nature prompted to evacuate them by stool or vomit; but if neither
follows

follows, (as in a clear body it may not) ballance your excefs next day with fafting, or a proportionable abftinence. This rule was very ftri&ly obferved by the Ancients, who thought it a great preventive to drink ftrong Wine once a month to that excefs, as fhould force nature to return it both wayes ; whereby they found that the fubtil heat of the Wine did colliquate their fuper-fluous humours, and referate obftrudions, and its impetuous fpirits evacuate the faid humours with the Wine; whereupon ufually followed a copious fweat, that procured a free tranfpiration ; which rule is to this day ftill kept in ufe among the *Germans.* How-ever I can in no wife approve of fo dange-rous a prefervative, that doth fo oft impell Drunkards into Feavers, burfting of a vein by vomiting, and inflammations of the Entrails.

The next of the *non naturals* is *Motion* and *Reft*; in which particular I would advife you to walk moderately(*ad Ruborem non fudorem*) until you be thorough hot, but not force your felf into a fweat; above all you muft be careful you come not in

P 3 the

the Summer from the Country out of that thin air into our thick mist in a great sweat, and open pores, into which our thick air intruding, may stop the pores, and occasion great Feavers, which too many are precipitated into, by their unadvised posting to Town in a sweat; This I suppose may be the reason, why those that return from *Naples* to *Rome* in the Summer, do undoubtedly fall into a Feaver.

In reference to their excretions, they must be sure to exonerate at least once a day; and if the dryness of their Guts be an obstacle in some hot and dry constitutions, they may remedy that by drinking a good draught of fresh small beer, or whey in a in a morning, and, feed upon laxative and moistning herbs, as boyl'd Spinnage, Lettice, Endive, &c.

What concerns their proportion of sleep, every one knows what his nature requires. But avoid sleeping after Dinner, or immediately after Supper; because it fills the head with fumes and vapours, and occasions Catarrhs.

In relation to the paſſions of the mind, take this ancient rule ; *Bene age, & latare,* i. e. Do well, and be cheerful. Avoid all occaſions of anger, fretting, and peeviſhneſs, which diſturb the blood, and enrage the corroſive humours. Thus much for the *Non Naturals.* Wee'l include one rule more ; conſidering that it's impoſſible, but the healthfulleſt perſon living in ſuch an air, and following the City mode in his Kitchen, muſt engender acrimonious humours, and obſtructions, and be ſubject to a conſtipation of the pores, it will prove very advantageous to open a Vein every Spring in caſe he be Plethorick, and purge ; or if only Cacochymick, to clarify his blood with a laxative ; and drink whey for a month or three weeks, to qualify the heat and ſharpneſs of his humours.

CHAP. XXXIV.

The Preservative for Consumptives.

THe *Preservative* part relates to the preventing of a Consumption in those that are inclined, or have lately conceived the seminaries of a Consumption. Who they are that are thus inclined, or are just entring the threshold of a Consumption, the foregoing discourse of Chap. 29. will acquaint you. In the *interim* take notice, that the same means we intend to prescribe for a cure, are likewise excellent preservatives, requiring only a moderation, according to the age of the Disease, time of year, and other circumstances.

The Indications taken from the *Non naturals*, which probably have made a great part of the first occasion of that Consumptive disposition, point at a mature change and rational correction of them.

1. The air appearing fo malicious in this Morbifique confpiracy, exacts a more particular regard. Wherefore it's of abfolute neceffity for Initiate Confumptives, to change that air how bad or good foever it may be reputed, wherein they have conceived or bred their confuming Seminaries; if bad, as thick, foggy miffy, fmoaky, moift, putrid, clowdy, or falin and acrimonious, they muft make choice of a ferene, thin, dry, temperate, fweet, and pleafant air; thus *Galen. lib.* 5. *Meth. Med.* advifed all tabefyed perfons, and fuch as were onely difpofed to a *Phthifis*, to remove to *Tabia*, a hilly place fituated between *Surrentum* and *Naples*, whofe temperature and drynefs of air, produced by the Sulphureous fmoaks of the Mount *Vefuvius* that's hard by to it, concurred to cure many a defperate Confumptive.

2. Though the air be generally experienced good, notwithftanding the Patient having contracted his evil there, poffibly by reafon of fome hidden contrariety that air harbours againft his temperament, is a fufficient indication for his changing the air, and

and that for a confiderable time, it may be a year, or two. For a moift Confumption the middle of *England* , as *Worcefterfhire,* *Glocefter,* or *Oxfordfhire,* feems to be en-rich'd with an air propitious for their reco-very ; however I imagine that fome places of *Languedock* one of the South Provinces of *France* , may for air excell that , or *Galen's Tabiæ*. For dry Confumptions a moifter air is more proper.

Neither is't only the change of air, that proves fo foveraign to Confumptives , but the change of Bread, Beer, Flefh, Com-pany and other circumftances , do very much conduce thereunto.

2. What advantage a loofe dyet imports to a healthful conftitution, the fame detri-ment it contributes to a declining or crazy one ; wherefore fince every fmall diftemper affumes fo eafie a growth from the leaft diforder of dyet, how much the more may a Confumptive difpofition, the worft of diftempers ; which certainly is an argument of the neceffity of a ftrict dyet, now here prefcribed to you in thefe rules.

1. Ab-

1. Abftain from all obftructive, melancholique, and dreggifh Victuals; as Beef,
Pork, Geefe, Ducks, Cheefe, Crufts of
Bread, Pyecruft, Pudding, Salt fifh, hard
boyl'd or fryed Eggs, or any kind of fryed
Meat. Likewife from hot Spices, as Pepper,
Ginger, Cloves, *&c.* and pickled meats,
as Anchiovy, Pickled Oyfters, or Her-
rings, Pickled Cowcumbers, *&c.*

2. Feed only upon meats of eafie digefture, and inclining fomewhat to a moift
temperature; as Veal, Chickens, Poulets,
Mutton, Lamb, Sweetbreads, Potch'd
Eggs, *&c.* and among the forts of Fifh,
Soals, Whitings, Perch, *&c.* among Herbs,
Lettice, Endive, Succory, Sorrel, Porcelain, Chervil, *&c.* but note that they muft
be boil'd.

3. Neither are you to allow your felf
flefh meat too liberally, becaufe according
to 2. *Aphor.* 11. *impure bodies the more you
feed them, the more you hurt them*; and
1. Aphor. 17. *When nourifhment is taken
beyond nature, it breeds a Difeafe*; becaufe
nature being oppreffed and diftemper'd,
cannot concoct the meats it affumes into
that

that temperate juice it doth when it's in better temper; but rather converts them all into ill humours, which must neceſſarily give an addition to thoſe Conſumptive ſalin corpuſcles; and beyond all others fleſh meat, as I have intimated before.

4. Dyet moſt upon Spoon meats, as Veal or Cock Broaths prepared with *French* Barly, Succory, Maiden hair, Agrimony, Graſs roots, Sweet Fennil, and Perſly roots, Raiſons and Dates.

Buttermilk affords a moſt Medicinal and Soveraign food in this diſeaſe. I remember I once knew a young Fellow at the *Hague*, who was fallen into an Ulcerous Conſumption upon ſpitting of blood, and notwithſtanding the danger of his Diſeaſe required the moſt potent Remedies, refuſed all help, and wholly devoted himſelf to Buttermilk, by which ſole dyet he recovered beyond the expectation of all that ſaw him: whence you may deduce of what conſequence a ſtrict dyet is.

5. Refrain from fleſh meat at ſupper, in lieu whereof you may now and then entertain your ſelf with a Pippin roaſted with
Saffron,

Saffron, and sweetned with Sugar of Roses, and *carui* Confects.

6. Drink no kind of strong Ale or Beer, or any liquor that contains Hops or Broom for its ingredients : but make use of small Ale brewed, out of an indifferent proportion of Malt, and a sufficient quantity of brown Sugar, in new river water, which excells that of the *Thames*. This makes the pleasantest and most delicate small liquor, proving very agreeable to the Palat and Stomach, and preventing Diseases. Most wines seem noxious, yet Rhenish Wines (I mean those small Wines, *Bachrach* and *Deal*) doth accidentally impinguate by helping the digesture, removing obstructions, and rendring the blood fluid and digestible. This is verifyed by the corpulent and fat habits of body of the Inhabitants of the *Rhine*, whom I observed all a long, in descending that river from *Bazil* in *Switzerland* as far as *Collen*, to be universally very fleshy, fat, and healthful; and my self, though entring into *Germany* in a lean case, was so much improved, before I left the *Rhine*, that in respect of corpulency

lency and fatnefs I differ'd little from any of them; which I could impute to nothing but their wine.

For *motion* obferve thefe rules. 1. Walk daily in a pleafant, airy, and umbragious Garden, Park, or Field. 2. Gentle travel in a Coach or on Horfeback through a healthful and divertifing countrey, doth oft conquer an initial Confumption. What concerns the Excretions and Retentions, and Paffions of the mind, regulate your felf according to former inftructions. Thefe prefcripts being thus obferved, we are to reflect upon indications drawn from internal caufes of growing extenuations; *viz.* the fubftraction of falin corrofive humours, engendred by the Spleen, and fublimed upwards by reafon of its obftructions. In this cafe the opening of the left *Median* in Plethoricks; afterwards the application of Leeches to the Hæmorrhoids; and hereupon a prefcription of a laxative and deoppilative whey, will anfwer all indications; and for particular derivatives, iffues, and lenitive Glyfters contribute great relief.

CHAP.

CHAP. XXXV.

The curative part for spitting of blood out of the Lungs.

HEre you are to diſtinguiſh, whether the Lung-vein be burſt; or corroded; or ſweats out blood; or gapes. The firſt of theſe indicates a ſudden evacuation of blood by *Phlebotomy*, for depletion and revulſion; and afterwards requires con-glütination. The ſecond indicates likewiſe a ſubtraction of blood in the beginning, for to revel and draw from the Lungs, and demulce the acrimony of the blood; and thereupon make uſe of conglutinating Me-dicines. The two latter indicate Phlebotomy for revulſion, reſtringents to ſtench, and incraſſatives to thicken the blood.

Wherefore at the firſt budding of this Symptom, eſpecially if a vein be burſted, and the ſpitting of blood copious, imme-diately evacuate as large a quantity of blood

blood out of the arm, as the Patient can bear without Swouning; for the greater and more sudden the evacuation is, the sooner the blood spitting stops; in which case expedition is very necessary, for otherwise the continual coughing would attract a greater stream of blood, and create a more difficult cure. So that Practick Authours advise ill, for subtracting blood in smaller proportions out of several veins at several times; which method, if the Patient cannot suffer the other, may notwithstanding be used, and seconded by Cupping-glasses applyed from below the shoulders downwards; likewise glysters, rubbing and tying of the extremities. Purgatives during the violence of the symptom are to be refrained; but afterwards, for to prevent its return, may be prescribed, and those only lenitives mixt with restringent purgatives; as *Myrobalans, Rhubarb,* &c. The other indications are to be answered out of these several *classes.*

Classis 1. Of ordinary conglutinatives and Emplasticks, *Cinquefoile, Tormentil, Millfoile, Cumpry, Willow weed,* &c.

Syrup

Syrup of Cumphry of Fernelius. The Emplasticks are *Bole armene, Terra sigillata Sanguis Draconis, spodium, gum Arabick, Dragant, Amylum* (or the finest kind of flower, where they make starch of) *Mastick, Franckincense,* &c. *Pyrola, Shepherds purse, Sanicle, Golden Rod.*

Cl. 2. Of Restringents. *Sumach, Plantain, Houseleek, Knotgrass, Mouse ear, Porcelain,* young *Oak Leaves, Vervaine, Horsetail, Ladies Bedstraw, Bramble bush Leaves, Speedwel, Acorn Caps, Pomgranat-shells, Red Roses, Wild Pomgranat-flowers, White Poppy seeds, Henbane Seeds, Myrtle Berries, Sumach Seeds, Coral, Blood Stone, Crabs shels burn'd, Rhubarb* tosted brown, *Acacia, Hypocistis, Crocus Martis, burn'd milk, Syrups of Dry Roses, Quinces, Myrtles, Porcelain, Poppies,* old conserve of *Roses,* &c. Out of these Physicians may form *Electuaries, Trochisces, Sublingual Pills, Apozems,* and distilled waters, according to their best thinking. To these wee'l subnect such as are more specifically recommended by famous Authours.

Q. *Trallianus*

Trallianus lib. 7. *cap.* 1. doth beyond all others, and that juftly extoll thefe following fpecifiques. 1. *The juices of Leeks and Netles, with a fmall quantity of Vineger, do moft egregiously ftop the blood of a burfted Vein.* 2. He tells us, *that the juice of Porcelain being drunk, is a moft excellent and powerful remedy.* 3. The decoction of *Cumfry root* is very much commended by him. 4. *The juice of Knotgrafs, doth fingularly conduce to any kind of fpitting of blood.* The fame vertue he attributes to the juice of *young Maftick leaves;* and particularly exprefles an efteem for *Sumach.* And beyond thefe formentioned Specificks he attributes an incomparable quality of cohibiting the moft defperate kind of bloody fputation, to a *Blood-ftone,* grinded upon a Porphyr to an impalpable powder, and exhibited in a dofe of Knotgrafs juice.

Galen 7. *de Comp.* *Med.* prefers white Henbane Seeds; but *Amatus Luf. Cent* 6. *car.* 4. fpeaks wonders of the juice of the greater fort of Nettles. *Hollerius lib.* 1. *cap.* 27. Sets a great efteem upon *Knotgrafs.*

grafs. *Duretius* writes a great praife of the
Diftill'd water of thofe tails that hang upon
Willow Trees. He puts likewife a great
confidence in *Trochifci è carabe.* *Valetius*
upon *Hol. exerc.* 27. recites a cure of one
that fpitted blood, who had tryed all the
famous Phyficians he could hear of, and at
laft was cured by *Scaliger,* who prefcribed
him this powder.

R. Spod, ros. rub. bol. arm. ter. figil.
hæmat. ã ʒ v. coral. rub. carab. margarit.
non perfor. ã ʒ ijſſ. gum. Arab. tragac.
ã. ʒ ij. Sem. papav. portul. fem. ros. rub.
fem. Arnoglos. corn. cerv. uft. ã ʒ iij.
Acac. fuc. Barb. hirc. fuc. glycyr. ã ʒ ij.
amyl. torrefact. ʒ j. M. f. Pulv. Dos. ʒ iij.
in aq. pluvial.

The fame prefcription he found afterwards extant in *Serap. cap.* 25. *tr.* 2. except that here is an addition of *coral. ear.*
and *Marg.*

Syr. è fymphyt. fernel. and Syr. coral.
quercet. are likewife in great requeft.
Iaterus writes he cured a Woman with
rochis. *Alkekengi cum opio* taken in
Goats milk. *Quercetan's Aq. ad Hæmoptyfin*

is much commended. Chymifts exhibit
9 or 10 drops of Oyl of Vitriol in the juice
of *Knotgrafs* ; they likewife make ufe of
Tincture, and *Salt of coral, crocus Martis,
ol. mart. tinct. Smaragd. ol. fuccin,* &c.
But beyond all thefe I prefer *Cerus. Antimon.* prepared with *Spirits of Vitriol*,
efpecially where there is fufpicion of coagulated extravafate blood, which may be
conjectured by the Feaver, faints, difficulty
of refpiration , and excretion of crumbs of
blood; in which cafe the Phyfician muft
look to his bufinefs, or elfe lofes his Patient.

    Galen prefcribed *oxycrate* to diffolve
the faid coagulated blood. Others commend *Pulv. carb. tiliæ, coagul. hædi, cer-
vi, leporis, fanguis hædi non concretu,
rad. rub. tinct. camphora, fperm. cæti, mumic,
ocul. cancror. cicer. rub. pulv. & Aq.
cherefal. Diaph. in peracut. Spir dulc. Merc.
effent. Bellid.* &c. But *Moufe-dung*
taken from one Scruple to half a dram in
chervil water excells them all.

    To return to the remainder of this Chap-
ter ; Thofe præcited Medicines proving
defective in ftenching that internal bleed-
in

ing, take your refuge to narcoticks, among
which that of *Halidæus* is moſt famous,
whereby he cured many in deſperate caſes, *viz.*

R. *Sem. Hyofcyam. papav. alb.* ā ℥ x.
terr. Sigil, coral. rubr. ā ℥ v. *Sacchar.
ros. vet. q. s. m. f. Elect. Dos.* ℥ j. *ad* ℥ j ſß
Mane & ſero. This compoſition *Crato* 5.
Epiſt. f. 377. aſſerts to be excerpted out of
Rhaſes his *Cont. Laudanum opiatum, pil.
cynoglos. Diacod. Pil. è ſtyrace, Philon.
rom.* may alſo be brought into uſe here.
In caſes of that importance, I would adviſe
Phyſicians not to loſe their time and op-
portunity in giving ſlight remedies, but
aſcend to thoſe more effectual Medicines.
The breaſt may be annointed with cool and
mild reſtrictives, as *Oyle of Roſes, Violets,
Myrtles,* &c. *Camphor* diſſolved in *Oxycrate* wherein clouts or rags being ſteeped
and applyed about the Teſticles, and
ſometimes about the waſte, are very
helpful. Iſſues in the Legs are moſt effective
in revelling the corroſive humours.

Galen ſuppoſing that ſometimes a diſtil-
lation of ſharp humours might corrode an

Ulcer

Ulcer into the Lungs, advifed a Confumptive Woman to fhave off her hair, and
apply an Emplafter of Piggeons dung, or
Thapfia, to extract, ablorb, and divert
thofe humours in the Brain; (others make
an iffue on the head at the *futura coronalis*
for the fame purpofe,) which kind of practice muft neceffarily rather add to the
Difeafe in attracting a greater quantity of
humours out of the whole to the head, afterwards falling down upon the removal of
the Emplafter in fuller ftreams to the Lungs
than before; befides fuch a kind of rough
Medicine being very diffonant to the dig-
nity and temperature of a noble part, might
infer irreparable dammages. But fince we
have made it vifible, that the brain is only
a *part tranfmittent*, and that humours oft
are precipitated to the Lungs, before they
arrive to that height of the brain, there can
no kind of benefit be expected from fo irra-
tional an application. On the other hand
thofe fubliming humours ought rather to be
intercepted before they are mounted to the
head, by *fublingual* Pils, *Trochifces*, ad-
ftringent and incraffating Syrups, *Lqochs*
Electua-

Electuaries, *&c.* To the fame intent *Celfus lib.* 3. *c.* 23. approves of exulcerations made under the Chin, on the Shoulders, Breaft, or Neck; *Hildanus* writes he cured feveral initial Confumptions chiefly by drawing a *Seton* through the Neck. When all is done, they do nothing, until they bend their defign and force to the *Part Mandant*, and eradicate the root of the Difeafe; which done, there remains nothing more.

The Patient is obliged to abftain from flefh; and dyet upon Panada, Rice Milk, Boyl'd Porcelain, Lettice, Potcht Eggs, *&c.* fome commend Pork, upon the anfwer of the Oracle, that advifed *Dumninus* the Philofopher to Hogs flefh, whereof as oft as he eated, his fpitting of blood ftop'd; and leaving it off, return'd; poffibly becaufe the juice of this fort of flefh is glutinous; for the fame reafon others approve of Eels, Mufcels, Cockles, Crabs, Lobfters, *&c. Damocrates* the Phyfician cured a *Roman* Woman only with Goats milk fed with Maftick-leaves. *Trallianus* relates, he cured feveral with Milk only.

Q 4   His

His drink ought to be a decoction of steel dust, burn'd Harts-horn, red Sanders, or Knotgrass, and sweetned with Sugar of Roses, dissolving in it besides a convenient quantity of *Sal Prunella*; or an Emulsion made of the four greater cold seeds, white Poppy seeds, and spirits of Vitriol. He must forbear much talk, walking, and all violent motions, and passions.

I'le only add an observation of a very speedy cure; one Mr. *S. D.* a Merchant, who through a violent vomit brake a Lung-vein; I caused immediately a large quantity of blood to be drawn out of his right Arm;& thereupon gave him this following

R. *Dulced. Mart. Spec. Hæmop. ā gr. 4. Opij Spag. præp. gr. ʃß Aq. urtic. Maj. ℥ ij. m. f. pot. capiat mane & sero.*

This he took thrice and was perfectly cured. The like effect it performed in one *W. S.* a Taylor.

CHAP.

CHAP. XXXVI.

The Cure of a Pulmonique Confumption.

THE Indications in the firft degree point at futable preparatives, to prepare thofe corrofive falin humours, and remove the forementioned obftructions of the Spleen, Stomach and Liver ; which is to be performed by *Agrimony, fumitory, Succory, Scabious, Borrage, Buglos, Endive, Maidenhair, Harts-tongue, Spleenwort, Cufcuta, Burnet, Grafs roots, ditch Dock roots, the five opening Roots, the four greater cold Seeds, Syr. e 5 rad. bizant. de cichor. cum Rh.* Some of thefe or all you may make ufe of in Whey, whereby having prepared thofe aduft humours, it's neceffary they fhould be purged by gentle purgatives and laxatives; as *Polypod. fem cartham. Manna, caffia, tamar. Syr. ros. fol. de Cichor. cum Rh, ros. fol. cum Agar. de pons.*

pom mag. de Epithym. Senna, Rhab. agar. crem. tart. Tart. vitriol &c. out of thefe you may compofe Apozems, to prepare the humours and at the fame time purge them; but by degrees (*per Epicrafin;*) after this if there was a fmall quantity of blood eva- cuated at the Hæmorrhoids by Leeches would be very advantageous. The cough in the mean while muft be remedied with Sy- rups, and Loochs, fublingual Pills and Trochifces to expectorate the humours out of the Lung-pipes. If the matter be tough thick and cleaving, it muft be cut, attenu- ated and deterged; if thin, it muft be thick- ned by incraffatives, as *Syr. Nymph. jujub. looch è Papav. portul.* &c. This kind of fhort cough in the firft degree is that which Phy- ficians call a *Tuffis Vulpina*, a Fox- cough. Touching the curative of the fecond degree, where we meet either with an Ulcer in Lungs, or an Ulcerous difpofition; the former, namely the Ulcer, muft be cleanfed or deterged, and afterwards cica- trized or confolidated. The firft is perform- ed by hot and dry Medicines; the latter by cold and dry. Moreover, there muft be a

par-

particular refpect had to the urgent fymptoms of this degree, *viz.* the Hectick Feaver
and Confumption of the parts. Having firft
fubtracted a part of the vitious humours,
by a laxative as *Manna, caffia, Syr. ros.
fol.* &c. it's generally agreed upon by the
moft famous ancient and modern Phyficians, that milk is the only Medicine and
food, that will anfwer all indications; for
by its wheyifh part it cleanfes and deterges;
by it's cheefy it conglutinates; by its
buttery part it reftores and nourifhes the
confumed parts; And by its unctuofity
promotes expectoration. But fince there
are feveral forts of milk, you are to make
diftinction of them. Womans milk is moft
nourifhing, but lefs detergent; Affes milk
is more cleanfing, and lefs reftorative; but
Goats milk is between both; that is, it's
more nourifhing and lefs cleanfing than
Affes milk, and more cleanfing and lefs
nourifhing than Womans milk. But becaufe
the cleanfing faculty is moft requifite,
Affes milk is univerfally preferr'd; and to
render it the more effectual, it's advifable to
feed the Affe with reftringent and detergent
herbs,

herbs, as Yarrow, Plantain, Vine leaves, Knotgrafs, Bramble-bufh leaves, &c. *Platerus* records feveral cured by Womans milk fuck'd warm out of the Breaft ; and among the reft there was one, that throve fo well with his Wives milk, that he purpofely got her with child again to prevent his want of milk for the future. Chamels milk is a degree beyond Affes for cleanfing. In ftead of Womans milk, Sheeps or Cows milk may be ufed. Likewife Mairs milk alone, or Cows milk being diluted with Whey, may be fubftituted in ftead of Affes or Chamels. Touching the ufe of milk, you muft obferve the quantity, time, and correction of it ; for the quantity, you muft accuftome your felf to it by degrees, beginning from a quarter of a pint, and afcending to a pint or a little more ; according to the parties appetite, and ftrength of digefture. The time muft be in the Mornings and Afternoons, taking your dofe alwayes five or fix hours before and after meat, warm from the Cow or Afs, and befure to refrain fleeping upon it, for otherwife it would fume up to the head.

Laftly,

Laftly, becaufe milk is fo apt to fowre in a weak Stomach, you muft fweeten it with Sugar of Rofes, or clarified Honey. Some boyl it with yolks of Eggs, to make it more nutritive ; others quench fteel in it to render it the more conglutinating.

But after all thefe *Encomia*, know that a milk dyet in many cafes proves hurtful, particularly, 1. When the body is affected with a putrid flow erratick, (difcernable, or fometimes latent) Feaver, as generally it is. 2. Confumptives are very fubject to evaporations and fumes flying to the Brain, obftructions of the Bowels, and difpofition to engender hot Cholerick and Salin humours ; all which evils milk is very apt to encreafe, nothing being more vaporous than it, nothing more Feaverifh, nothing more obftructive, by reafon of its cheefy parts, and nothing more convertible into hot cholerick humours than it's buttery parts, as appears in Children, whom it doth fo extremely fill with green and yellow gall, and fleam ; and difpofes them to Catarrhs, Confumptions, Feavers, Loofeneffes, &c. 3. Moft Phyficians forbid

bid milk to those, that are troubled with weak Stomachs, sowre Belchings, Grumblings in their Guts (*Borborygmi*) Loosenesses, all which Consumptives are seldom free from. 4. Many passages of *Hip.* do also disuade 2. *Aphor.* 11. and 17. and *lib. de vet. Med. Meat eaten in too great a quantity tabefies the body*, and *lib. de. loc. in hom. If the body doth not digest the meat it eats, it's rendred lean*; besides several other places, which would prove too tedious to recite. Wherefore you must be very careful, you do not exceed in your milk dyet; but the surest way is not to meddle with it without a Physicians advice. Moreover take away the root and cause of the Consumption, and the body will soon thrive upon it.

For these reasons I do attribute much more to a Whey dyet, which I have advised to many, with the greatest success imaginable, enjoyning them to drink nothing but white Whey sweetned with Sugar or old Conserve of Roses; to Dine and Sup upon Buttermilk, boyl'd with French Barly beaten in a Mortar, or Oat-meal, and afterwards

wards fweetned with Sugar of Rofes, and coloured yellow with *Englifh* Saffron. But left they fhould be clyed with that, they may gratifie their Palats with variety of Broaths, and efpecially with Broath made of an old Cock, with the addition of aperitive and pulmonique herbs, which together with the ufe of fome laxatives only, is in great vogue among the *Italian* Phyficians for the cure of Confumptions. Some advife their Patients to dyet upon Crabs, Lobfters, Oyfters, Cockles, Mufcels, Frogs, &c. but againft reafon, thofe meats being of too hard a digefture for weak Stomachs; neverthelefs the juices expreffed out of them, or liquors diftilled from them, are experienced very proficuous. Others prefcribe milk boyl'd with flower, thick ptifan, confections out of Capons, Partridge, and Tortifes flefh, Crabs, Lobfters, Sweet Almonds, Piftaches, White poppy feeds, the four greater cold Seeds, &c. For their ordinary drink, they approve of Barly Water, Small Meetheglin, the decoction of Hartshorn, or the Small Ale defcribed in Chap. 34. But beware of ftale Beer.

The

The Air ought to be dry and temperate; witness the story of that old Woman, that was preserved many years by the dry Air of the Bakers Oven, where she was used to work. *Aretæus* commends a Sea Air, and therefore the Ancient Physicians were wont to send their Patients to *Alexandria*, for to have the benefit of the Salt Air during the Voyage, which being of a drying nature, they conceived might conduce to the drying up of the Ulcer in the Lungs. But in my opinion the Sea Air being nauseous, moving one to Vomit, and stirring the humours of the body, should rather prove offensive. *Pliny* doth highly esteem the Air of Forests, where pitch is collected.

The detersives for the Ulcer are composed out of Vulneraries, agglutinatives, and pectorals; viz. *Burnet, Centaury, Betony, Agrimony, Vervain, Mouse-ear, Avens, Ladies Mantle, Arsmart, Periwincle, Bugle, Lilly of the Valley, Solomon's Seal, Serpentine, Snakeweed, Aristol. rot. Cicer. rubr. Isop, Water Germander, Colts-foot, Card. Benedict. Lung-wort, Maiden hair, Scabious, Penny-royal, Ground Ivy, Cud-*
weed,

weed, *Ros solis*, *Origan*, *Horehound*, *Oak of Jerusalem*, *Calamint* , *St. Johns-wort*, *Elicampaine*, *Squils*, *Orris*, *Myrrh*, *Terebinthih*, *Fox Lungs*, *Spec. diaireos*, *Diacalaminthe*, *Looch San. & expert. è pulm. vulp. Syr. nicot. è ped. cat.* &c. The agglutinatives we have set down in the Chapter preceding, and are to be made use of when the Ulcer is sufficiently cleansed. The experience of famous Practitioners recommends to us several Specifiques. 1. *Ros solis* is extold above most other Pulmonicks by several. 2. *Speed-well* is likewise very frequently used against Ulcers in the Lungs; an Herb certainly without comparison. 3. *Camerarius* speaks much in the praise of *Oak of Jerusalem*; which also makes the *basis* of *Syr. Botryos*, described in the *Lond. disp.* 4. The generality of Physicians attest *Spotted Lungwort* to be a most egregious Pulmonique, both for deterging and conglutinating an Ulcer in the Lungs. 5. An ingenious Physician at *Padua* told me this following for a great secret in an Ulcerous Consumption of the Lungs. *Masterwort-root* boyl'd in Metheglin, and afterward

R   mix'd

mix'd with a third part of *aq. Sperm ranar.*
6. *Langius* and others make ule of *Ground
Ivy,* for the laſt and extreme remedy. You
may take it either deſtilled, in the Juyce,
or Syrup; diſſolving only in them ſome
Conſerve or Suggar of Roſes. 7. *Saffron* is
commonly-ſtiled the ſoul of the Lungs,
which when they are ready to be ſtifled and
choak'd with thick tough ſteam and purulent matter, have been miraculouſly recovered by a doſe of Saffron in wine; wherefore no preſcription for Pulmoniques ought
to paſs without ſome grains of Saffron in it.
8. *Millepedæ* or Palmers have for many
Ages been reputed the greateſt deterſives
and cleanſers of the Lungs, a quantity of
them being tyed in a fine Linnen rag, and
ſteeped in Metheglin or Whey, and ſo uſed;
or being burned to aſhes in an oven and
mixed with old Conſerve of Roſes. 9. *Avicen. lib. 3. Fen. 10. Tract. 5. cap. 5.
meſues. cap. de Phthiſi. Valleriola lib. 5.
Obſ. 5. Foreſt. libr. 16. Obſ. 58. Montan.
in Conſ. 152.* do all bring in unqueſtionable
Teſtimonies of ſeveral, by them particularly
mentioned, deſperate Conſumptives, perfectly

fectly cured of deep and sordid Ulcers in the Lungs, by the sole means of Suggar of Roses; but of at least a year old, & devoured in great quantities several times in a day, and so continued for some weeks. 10. *Fonseca consult.* 58. *tom.* 1. sets a great value upon the Decoction of yellow Sanders. 11. *Arcaus lib. de Febr. Erastus lib.* 3. *Conf.* 8. *Fracast. lib.* 3. *de morb. contag. cap* 8. *Ingrassias in consult. pro sist. pect. Stabelius in Disput,* and several others, recite a great number of Phthisical cures, and those desperate ones, performed by a Decoction of *Guaiacum* wood. 12. *Trallianus lib* 7. *c.* 1. speaks wonders of the use of Bloodstone. *Cardan* writeth no less of the Decoction of Crabs Legs and Tails; *Fern.* of the Syrup of Cumphry, others of the Syrup of *St. Johnswort flowers,* and *Syrup of Tobacco.* 12. For Compositions, this following powder of *Haly Abbas* is by *Valescus, Forestus, Rondeletius,* and all others received for a singular Medicine, whereby the three former cured some Consumptives, beyond their own expectation. R. *Sem. pap. alb.* ℥x. *gum. arab. amyl.* ã ℥iij *sem portul.*

R 2 *malv.*

malv. alth. ā ʒ v. sem. cucurb. cucum. citrul.
cydon. ā ʒ vij. Spod. glycyr. gum. tragac.
ā ʒ iij. m. f. Pulv. 14. This of *Trallianus*
I esteem equal with the best composition
that ever was prescribed by any. R. Suc.
sempervivi. passi cretici, mel. attic. ℥. cyath.
2. sem. attic. cucum. sativ. cupres. ā ʒ j.
coq. ad Consump. med. part. Colat. adde pic.
liq. cyath. ℥ coq. ad consist. mellis ; huic
admisce nard. syriac. ʒ j. thuris ʒ iij. Croci,
pip. alb ā ʒ ij. m. f. Elect.

Here I have registred to you the most
efficacious Medicines of this and the former
ages, which unless applyed by a dexterous
hand, may sooner kill than cure. Moreover
note these detersives may be mixt with the
restringents, consolidatives, & incrassatives
of the preceding Chapter, according as the
Patients condition shall require.

For external means, drying suffumiges or
smoaks are oft prescribed with good success.
They are usually composed out of *Frankin-
cense*, *Myrrh*, *Pitch*, *Olibanum*, *Benzoin*,
Styrax. *Gum*. *hedera*, *Amber*, *Rose leaves*,
Coltsfoot dryed, *Sanders*, *lign*. *Aloes*, &c.
but the fume of *Sandaracha* is particularly
com-

ommended. Emollient & temperate Oyls
& Liniments seem to facilitate respiration,
which the Physician must alwayes have an
ye to, and therefore it's necessary he should
ver mix some lenient pectorals with his
ther Medicines : Issues in the lower parts
to also divert.

Hermetical Physicians go another way to
work; they begin with a galliard vomit, and
to proceed to detersives and agglutinatives;
*viz. Flowers of Brimstone, Balsam and milk
of Sulphur, Elixir proprietatis, cryftal mart.
Extract. Ariftol. rot. spir. salis dulc. Ol.
vitriol, ol. mercur. dulce, spir. sulphuris per
camp. ol. succin. magift. ocul. cancror. magift.
perlar. tinct. sal. & magift. coral. rub. sacchar. satura. Mynfighti. antimon. diaphor.*

To Dogmatifts this Chymical practice
seems suspicious; in regard that vomits do
violently conquaffate the Lungs, and tare
the Ulcer wider. Moreover *Hip. 4. Aph. 8.*
doth very much condemn vomits in such,
as are onely disposed to a *Phthisis,* much
more in those that are already tabefyed.
Hereunto may be replyed, that vomits
though they infer some small detriment to
the

the Lungs, yet they import a far greater
benefit by working immediately upon the
parts mandant ; and *Hip.* himself *lib. 2. de
Morb.* did frequently exhibit *Hellebor* to
Confumptives, which is experienced to be
a very churlith Medicine.

On the other hand Chymifts quarrel
with Dogmatifts for letting blood in Confumptions, where nature is already fo much
defrauded of its *Genius*, and confequently
rather hungers for a greater fupply of
nutriture : this objection they eafily anfwer, in afferting that in many Confumptives there is a *Plethora ad vires*, (though
in no wife *ad vafa*) a great acrimony in
their blood, and an impetuous afflux of
humours to their Lungs, which do very
urgently indicate Phlebotomy ; whereby
Hipp. 5. *Epid.* 6. recovered a Confumptive, whofe difeafe contemned all other
remedies ; and *Galen* 6. *Epid.* cured a
Woman of a *Fhthifis* by the fame means.
Several other Authours likewife obferve
many refcued from imminent Confumptions by detracting fmall proportions of
blood. No doubt but Phlebotomy and
Vomits

Vomits have their ufe in this malady; but the Temperament, Age, Sex, and *Idiofyn-crafia* of the Patient, degree of the Difeafe, and other urgent or contraindicating fymp-toms muft be exquifitely obferved.

It's time I fhould take leave of my Rea-der, which the urgency of my affairs doth now prompt me to ; However for his laft farewel we'l entertain him with fome few obfervations of mixt cures, namely partly fpagyrical, and partly dogmatical.

Obf. 1. One *G. T.* a Merchant's Appren-tice, upon a continuated debauch, was fur-prized with a tedious Cough, oft expectora-ting fmall quantities of blood, whereupon he foon dropt into a proper Confumption, but was in a fhort time recovered by thefe means; I advifed him to the Country, where by my appointment a proportion of blood was extracted twice out of the Hæmorrhoids by Leeches. Before and afterwards was feve-ral times purged with this bole. *R. extract. rec. cafs.* ℥ *ſß pulp. tamarind. man. calabr.* ã ʒij. *cryftal tart.* Ðj. *Rhab el. pu. v. agar. rec. troch.* ã Ð *ſß ſpic. nard. gr.* 4. *cum facchar.*

M. P.

M. F. Bol. for sixteen dayes he took this Elect. mornings and evenings, drinking upon it a draught of Decoct. of red Sanders sweetened with Sugar of Roses, and acuated with a drop or two of Spir. *Sulphur. per camp. R. Magist. stypt. Specif. Hect. croc. angl. ã gr.* 4. *Conserv. ros. vet.* ℥ j.

M. F. Bol. His ordinary drink was white Whey; his dyet broaths alter'd with herbs, and oftimes Buttermilk.

Obs. 2. A young woman aged 24, spitting blood and matter upon the stoppage of her courses, was let blood out of the foot, and oft purged with *Diaprunum lenit.* ℥ ß *Merc. dulc. gr.* 15. *crem. tart.* Ð j. She drank a decoct. of *Sarsa* with *Veron. agrimon. heder. ter. Dates, Corrents,* and *Liquorish* for 21 dayes, at the expiration of which term she was cured of her Cough, and there appeared a shew of her flowers. I advised her also to *Looch. Papap.* and *è Pulm. vulp.* ana. and to make an Issue in her left Leg.

Obs. 3. A Child aged 3. deform'd with the Rickets, & consumed to skin and bones, was cured in a month by the *Tincture* of tartar,

tartar, taking two drops twice or thrice a day in Whey.

Obs. 4. I have seen many thousands of Diseased in the Hospitals of *France, Germany, Italy, Holland, Flanders,* and other parts, but never observed so many great Diseases complicated in one body, as not long since in one of my Patients; the party had been seised of a latent venereal malady two or three years together, and newly again surprized with a Green virulent Gonorrhe, a constant excretion of purulent matter; an immitigable Cough, a confirm'd Dropsie, a most sordid Ulcer in the Kidneys, evacuatting constantly a great quantity of blood and *Pus* (matter) with his Urin, a perfect Consumption, great obstructions of his Bowels, and many other most urgent Symptoms. Whence I could observe the strange force of nature, though in a body naturally weak, to support such a number of great Diseases; and that which to me appeared more strange, was an intermission of at least two pulsations in nine or ten, continuing that type for several hours, I am confident, if not dayes.

Obs. 5.

Obf. 5. A Smith that had expectorated putrid, thick, ugly matter for at least two months, I cured out of charity; I gave him two *dofes* of *Antimon. refufcit.* the preparation whereof I have divulged to you in *Venus Unmask'd*; and advifed him to drink twice a day a fmall draught of Spring water being render'd bitter with foot burn'd out of wood, and fweetned again with brown Sugar, which in a month perfectly cured him. I thought to have prefented you with feveral other remarques; but that the Bulk of this Treatife being already fwell'd beyond my purpofe, obliges me to come to an

E N D.

The Table of Contents.

CHAP.

The Table of Contents.

CHAP

The Table of Contents.

CHAP.

The Table of Contents.

of

The Table of Contents.

FINIS.

Lightning Source UK Ltd.
Milton Keynes UK
UKOW04f2008280617

304283UK00002BA/20/P